The Dignity of Human Procreation and the Simple Case in Vitro Fertilization

Patrick Idoko Abem

The Dignity of Human Procreation and the Simple Case in Vitro Fertilization

Moral-Theological Debate in the Light of "Donum Vitae"

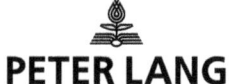

Lausanne • Berlin • Bruxelles • Chennai • New York • Oxford

Library of Congress Cataloging-in-Publication Data
A CIP catalog record for this book has been applied for at the Library of Congress.

Bibliographic Information published by the Deutsche Nationalbibliothek
The Deutsche Nationalbibliothek lists this publication in the Deutsche Nationalbibliografie; detailed bibliographic data is available online at http://dnb.d-nb.de.

ISBN 978-3-631-89310-4 (Print)
E-ISBN 978-3-631-89676-1 (E-PDF)
E-ISBN 978-3-631-89677-8 (E-PUB)
10.3726/b20545

© 2023 Peter Lang Group AG, Lausanne
Published by Peter Lang GmbH, Berlin, Deutschland

info@peterlang.com - www.peterlang.com

All rights reserved.

All parts of this publication are protected by copyright. Any utilisation outside the strict limits of the copyright law, without the permission of the publisher, is forbidden and liable to prosecution. This applies in particular to reproductions, translations, microfilming, and storage and processing in electronic retrieval systems.

This publication has been peer reviewed.

*Dedicated to Infertile Couples
and
Those Who Work to Promote the Dignity of Human Procreation*

Preface

This publication, *The Dignity of Human Procreation and the Simple Case In Vitro Fertilization: Moral-theological Debate in the Light of "Donum Vitae,"* is the fruit of an academic research completed in 2015 on the moral and theological debate regarding the Simple Case in vitro fertilization (IVF). The focus of the research was basically limited to the theological and moral debate among some Catholic scholars who sustain that, unlike the regular IVF, the procedure of homologous extra-corporeal human fertilization is not complicated with ethical issues. It is believed that in this technique there is no use of donor gametic cells and precautions are taken to fertilize only the number of eggs that are intended to be transferred to the womb of the woman to avoid intentional destruction of excess embryos. However, in the light of Catholic Magisterium, the Simple Case IVF does not meet the requirement for the dignity of human procreation and so remains a problematic medical procedure for the generation of a new human life. This magisterial position has met discordant reception among some Catholic moral theologians after the publication of *Donum Vitae* in 1987.[1] While some scholars welcomed and appreciated the moral evaluation and conclusion of the document, some dissented. It is the desire to present the synthesis of the different positions to a wider readership that this current publication has become relevant. Hence, the basic goal of this publication is to offer a sound moral evaluation and guidance regarding medical techniques in human procreation with reference to the so-called Simple Case IVF.

Since 2015 when our dissertation was completed, there might have been improvements in new reproductive technologies to achieve more efficient success but the moral arguments of Catholic scholars on the Simple Case IVF have remained the same. At this moment there is no available known update on official Catholic moral teaching to suggest that the Simple Case IVF has become a licit means to generate human life. The reason for this

---

1 Congregation for the Doctrine of the Faith, *Instruction Donum Vitae, On Respect for Human Life in Its Origin and On the Dignity of Human Procreation*, 22 February 1987: in *AAS* 80 (1988).

position borders on the dignity of human life and the sacredness of marriage which the procedure does not uphold by its very nature and meaning. Whereas, almost all Catholic moral theologians and ethicists do not have many problems receiving the negative judgment of *Donum Vitae* on heterologous artificial insemination and regular IVF as procedures of generating human life, only some find it difficult and unacceptable for the Simple Case IVF to be proscribed because they consider it less problematic. The Catholic Scholars who express dissent against the evaluation and conclusion of the Magisterium on the Simple Case seem to suggest that the destruction of human embryos and use of a donor constitute the only problem of this procedure. But their reasoning can be considered inadequate because it fails to understand the theological and moral basis for the dignity of human procreation. The fact that the Simple Case IVF violates the principle of inseparability of the conjugal act by seeking the generation of human life outside of the conjugal act makes it intrinsically illicit. A medical procedure can only meet the moral requirement of human procreation when it assists the conjugal act and not when it substitutes as in the case of the Simple Case IVF. The destruction of human embryos, selective abortion, use of donor, etc., are equally ethically problematic in addition to replacing the conjugal act. Since 1978 which occasioned a remarkable leap in reproductive technology with the birth of Joy Louis Brown by means of IVF, the world has not remained the same. The production of human embryos *in vitro* has posed many challenges of both legal and moral dimensions. These challenges are also found with the so-called Simple Case IVF and that is the reason the current work is important for providing the different moral and theological perspectives that are required for the right choice or rejection of a medical technique to assist infertile couple have a child. The moral position of the Church sustains that the technique for generating a child must respect the conjugal act by assisting it to achieve its end and not replacing it.

The gift of a child brings delight to couples as they find in their children the fruitfulness of their marital love. Children in turn strengthen the bond of marital love and in many cases, the children become a kind of security to marital bond of parents. This does not mean that the validity of marriage comes from marital fecundity. No, the validity of marriage comes from the consent of the couple.² In many homes, couples who have not heard the cry of a baby in their marriage, suffer a lot of taunt, maltreatment and disrespect from neighbors and in-laws. Some spouses even suffer same from their partners. We can testify to the broken and breaking marriages around us for the simple reason of childlessness. We cannot deny the sad cases of marital infidelity in contemporary society bordered on the alleged need for seeking a child or as means of testing one's fertility or as a fallout of frustration with partners for not being able to have a child. In the age of advancements in medical science and technology, it has become possible to have a child by medical means other than the conjugal act. Undoubtedly, the importance of a child in marriage cannot be overemphasized and the pains of childlessness in marriage cannot be underrated. That is why, it seems legitimate and understandable to find couples seek medical means, including bypassing the conjugal act, the sole sanctuary for generating human life, to producing human embryos in the laboratory. For the fact that it is possible to have a child through these artificial means does not make such decisions or means morally right. Science should be used as a gift to enhance human dignity and not otherwise.

In Catholic moral reasoning, it is not acceptable that an action which intrinsically violates human dignity becomes morally acceptable because of circumstance and intention. This is the problem with the Simple Case IVF. In the impressive work published in July 2018 to celebrate the forty years of IVF, Heather E. Ross and Guido Pennings established that the legal and ethical concerns which previously surrounded IVF "have died down to make for the recognition that surplus embryos and embryos destruction were an inevitable part of IVF. This is remarkable since the main reasons for creating more embryos than necessary [meaning: more than could be replaced in the fresh cycle] were pragmatic. In fact, it would have been possible [and still is] to practice IVF without violating the rule of respect for human life in the form of embryos."³ These authors have acknowledged

---

2 *Code of Canon Law* (1983), Canon 1057§ 1
3 Heather E. Ross and Guido Pennings, "Legal and Ethical Aspects of In Vitro Fertilization," in Craig Niederberger and Anthony Pellicer (eds.), *Forty Years of IVF* (American Society for Reproductive Medicine, Elsevier Inc., 2018), 299–300: Forty-years-of-IVF_2018_Fertility-and-Sterility.pdf, checked on October 23, 2022.

that in the history of IVF, aspects of disrespect for human life have been part of its practice and that is why it the Simple case IVF remains ethically problematic. However, Ross and Pennings believe that IVF could also be practiced without destroying human embryos, the indication that points to the Simple Case. Despite the improvement that can be made to forestall the creation of excess embryos and destruction of leftovers, the very nature of this procedure entails achieving fertilization as the result of a laboratory experiment and not as the fruit of personal sexual union of the couple and for this fact, the procedure violates the dignity of human procreation. In fact, no recent research on the theological and moral aspects of the Simple Case of IVF published after 2015 of our research, has contradicted our negative judgment of the procedure in the light of the Instruction *Donum Vitae*. There are other means of medically assisted procreation that are morally acceptable and recommended for couples who have difficulty in achieving conception naturally. For instance, the Natural Procreative Technology (NaPro Tech) and similar technologies which assist the conjugal act to achieve procreation have been recommended as alternatives to any form of in vitro fertilization. This work does not claim to have exhausted all aspects of this subject, but it is the first of its kind to articulate in a volume the debate of some Catholic Scholars on this theme. It is therefore to be considered a modest contribution that can provide a moral guidance and of stimulating thoughts for further investigations.

Acknowledgments

I would like to acknowledge and express gratitude to God and to all persons who I consider to be responsible for the success of this dissertation. First and foremost, let me echo the words of the psalmist to recognize that success comes pre-eminently from God: "If God does not build a house in vain do its builders toil. If God does not guard a city in vain does it guard keep watch" (Psalm 127,1). Therefore, if God did not grant His help, in vain would have been our efforts to bring this study to a successful end. To Him the all-knowing and Divine Trinity, the giver of life with whom every good gift comes, I remain eternally indebted for His guidance in the course and completion of this research project.

To my former Bishop, Most Rev. Dr. John E. Ayah, currently, the Diocesan Bishop of Uyo and Apostolic Administrator of the diocese of Ogoja, who granted me the privilege and the means to undertake further studies in Rome, I give my respectful and sincere gratitude. Indeed, he enjoys a special place in my heart as father and motivator in my priestly life and in the realization of this work. I equally express my gratitude to the priests of the Catholic diocese of Ogoja, Nigeria, whose fraternal encouragements and prayers have accompanied me all these years of studies in Rome. Special thanks go to the respectable fraternity of Ogoja student-priests in Rome: Frs. Stephen Apebende, Kenneth Odibu and Fidelis Kajibia, their moral support has been amazing. Other brethren, Frs. Joe-Martins Ojeka, Joe-Macus Ogan, Josephat Ekor, Patrick Okuta, Mark Binang, Kenneth Inaku Egere, Basil Ejim, Victor Dakwan, George Adaje, Paul Okora and Peter Egbonyi have played various remarkable roles, I owe them my gratitude.

And to my respectable Moderator, Prof. Dr. Pablo Requena Meana, words are obviously inadequate to render my unalloyed appreciation for his extraordinary demonstration of patience, kindness, guidance and encouragement during this study. I equally heartily thank the second Moderator, Prof. Dr. Martin Schlag, whose inputs in this work remain remarkable. To the Administration and Staff of the Pontifical University of the Holy Cross (Santa Croce), Rome, I extend my profound affection and thanks. I thank in a special way the Dean of the faculty of Theology, Rev. Mons. Angel

Rodríguez-Luño and the Staff of this faculty for their inspiration and commitment to work that I have benefited immensely.

My appreciation equally goes to the Scholarship Boards of the Papal Foundation and the *Centro Académico Romano Fundacion* (CARF) of whose goodwill I was granted scholarship for my Licentiate and Doctorate programs respectively. I remain grateful to the Personnel of the Students' Consultation Office of Santa Croce, for their support in my studies. I acknowledge the spiritual assistance of Frs. Cristian Mendoza, Antonio Rodríguez Rivera and Antonio Porras, how could it have been without their friendship!

To the Nigerian Priests, Religious and Seminarians in Rome, I remain appreciative of the encouragement I received to get this study completed. I acknowledge with affection and express my gratitude to the Sisters of the Congregation of the Daughters of Mary Mother of Mercy in Rome, who were always praying for God's mercies for me and for the success of this work. In a special way I would like to express my indebtedness of gratitude to Frs. Cosmas Oscar Ekwere, Anthony Naah, Martín Miguel Astudillo, Emmanuel Faweh, Valentine Onwunjiogu, Alex Ogbanufe, ThankGod Okafor, Lawrence Ezike, Joseph Ediae, Augustine Okon, Louis Mary Ocha, and Srs. Christine Mary Ugobi, Eugenia Dinneya, Ogechi Nwagwu, Genevieve Egan, Gloria Agbor, Josephine Ngede, Maris Sylvia, Vivien Anukanti, Rose Oko, Rose Abang, Patricia Oko and Theresa Ashi, for their friendship and love which sustained my effort in this work.

I cannot fail to acknowledge and thank my cherished friends at the Pontifical Filipino College, Rome, where I took residence for two academic years. In the same token of gratitude, I express a million thanks to the Congregation of the Figlie della Provvidenza per le Sordomute, whose house I stayed to complete this program. In a similar manner, I am particularly thankful to the Personnel of the library of Immaculate Heart Seminary, Huntington, NY, USA and the Human Life International Library, Rome, Italy, for their cordial and generous permission to use their facilities for my research. Many thanks equally go to the late Dr. William E. May, who read my project proposal and gave his encouragement. May God grant him eternal peace! I am also grateful to Frs. James Akpan, Francis Afu, Ashley Beck and Sr. Mary Ijechukwu who proofread some parts of this work and made useful suggestions.

Acknowledgments

I remember with affection and gratitude the encouragements of the Parishioners of San Giovanni Battista, Genova and Santissimo Crocifisso, Belmonte, Palermo, where I spent some holidays for pastoral experiences. And to the Parishioners of St. Patrick's Church, Bay Shore, New York, I owe special thanks. The hospitality I enjoyed in this parish during my summer vacations accorded me a great deal of assistance to work on this project. I am heartily grateful to Msgr. Thomas Coogan and Josephine Cahill with the personnel of this parish for arranging a library for me to study and for my upkeep. I extend my profound appreciation to my friends in the parishes of St. Raphael's Church, East Meadow and Sacred Heart Church, Hartsdale, New York, USA. I remember with deep sense of joy and gratitude the benevolence of my brothers and friends Frs. Cyril Bayim, Philip Tah, Noel Effiong MSP and Christopher Okoli. My special appreciation goes to Angela Hsi for her overwhelming support in this project.

With unquantifiable sense of appreciation, I acknowledge the support of my parents, Mr. Stephen Abem Akpikpe and Mrs. Cecilia Ilufu Ibam. Together with them in this rite of gratitude are my siblings and extended family members both natural and Christian. I acknowledge especially the support of Sir and Lady Patrick Akwaji, Lady Felicia Ogar, Sir and Lady Effenji Odey, Andrew Achi and Joseph Oshie.

The list of persons who are deserving of my acknowledgement and gratitude is endless, but to one and all, I appreciate every bit of the goodwill and kind gesture I received to get this project accomplished.

Ad Maiorem Dei Gloriam!!!

Table of Contents

Preface 7

Acknowledgements 11

Table of Contents 15

List of Abbreviations 21

General Introduction 23
   1. The Actual Problem 25
   2. The Main Argument 26
   3. Objectives and Doctrinal Relevance of This Project 28
   4. Methodology and Delimitation of the Work 30
   5. Organization of Chapters 32

Chapter One The Magisterium and Some Theological Opinions on Artificial Procreation 35
   Introduction 35
   A. Magisterial Teachings on Artificial Procreation Prior to *Donum Vitae* 38
      1.1. The Teaching of Pius XI: *Casti Connubii*, 31 December 1930 38
      1.2. The Teaching of Pius XII 41
         1.2.1. Address to the International Congress of Catholic Medical Doctors, 29 September 1949 42
         1.2.2. Allocution to the Italian Catholic Union of Midwives, 29 October 1951 45
         1.2.3. Allocution to Participants at the Second World Congress on Infertility and Sterility, 19 May 1956 47

  1.2.4. Allocution to Participants at the Seventh International Congress of Haematology, 12 September 1958 50
 1.3. The Teaching of Paul VI: *Humanae Vitae*, 25 July 1968 ... 51
 1.4. Opinions of Some Theologians 53

B. An Overview of the Instruction *Donum Vitae* 61
 1.1. The Instruction's Three Lines of Argument against Artificial Fertilization 61
  1.1.1. The Principle of Inseparability of the Conjugal Act 62
  1.1.2. The "Language of the Body" Argument 66
  1.1.3. The "Begotten-Not-Made" Argument 69
 1.2. Moral Principles of *Donum Vitae* 71
  1.2.1. The Life of the Human Being 71
  1.2.2. Marriage as the Only Licit Context for Procreation 73
  1.2.3. The Dignity of Human Procreation 75
  1.2.4. Biomedical Technology as a Gift in the Service of Life 76
  1.2.5. *Donum Vitae* on the Simple Case IVF-ET 78
  1.2.6. Relationship between Moral and Civil Law 83

Synthesis of the Chapter 85

Chapter Two Moral-Theological Arguments in Favor of the Simple Case of Homologous IVF-ET 89

Introduction 89

A. The Critique of *Donum Vitae* 91
 1.1. An Overview of Its Argumentation against the Instruction 91
 1.2. Narrowness in Its Range of Consultation 93
 1.3. The Alleged Physicalism or Biologism of *Donum Vitae* 98
  1.3.1 Adequate Consideration of the Human Person ... 100

Table of Contents

      1.3.2   Hierarchy of Values of the Human Person 105
      1.3.3   The Body as Instrument of the Human Person 108
  1.4.   Inadequate Use of Its Natural Law Methodology 111
  1.5.   Summary 114

B. On the Conjugal Act and Its Understanding by the
Dissenting Theologians 115
  1.1.   An Overview 115
  1.2.   On the Principle of Totality and the Conjugal Act 117
  1.3.   On the Moral Object and the Principle of
         Inseparability of the Conjugal Act 122
  1.4.   On the Doctrine of Double Effect and
         the Conjugal Act 129
  1.5.   Summary 132

C. Begotten-not-Made 134
  1.1.   An Overview 134
  1.2.   The Simple Case IVF-ET as Life Enhancing 136
  1.3.   The Simple Case IVF-ET Technology Accords with
         Human Dignity 137
  1.4.   The Simple Case as an Imperfect Act Not an Immoral
         Act 139
  1.5.   Summary 140

Synthesis of the Chapter 142

Chapter Three   In Defense of *Donum Vitae*'s Arguments against the Simple Case of Homologous IVF-ET 143

Introduction 143

A. The Anthropological Argumentation of *Donum Vitae* 144
  1.1.   An Overview of the Argumentation Methodology 144
  1.2.   Argument Based on the Natural Law 146
  1.3.   The Unity of the Human Person Adequately
         Considered 153

	1.4.	The Human Role in Procreation and the Logic of *Donum Vitae*	157
	1.5.	On the Moral Object of the Simple Case IVF-ET	163
	1.6.	Summary	174

B. The Dignity of Human Procreation 175
    1.1. An Overview of the Argument on the Dignity of Human Procreation 175
    1.2. The Unitive-Procreative Significance of the Conjugal Act 176
    1.3. The Conjugal Act: Its Unity and Plenitude 183
    1.4. The Conjugal Act: A Personal Act of the Couple 187
    1.5. Summary 191

C. The Child Is Begotten, Not Made 192
    1.1. An Overview of the Argument 192
    1.2. The Child as a Gift of God in Marriage 193
    1.3. An Instrumental Logic of Productivity Implied in the Technology 198
    1.4. The Child Is Not a Means of Fulfilling Parents' Desire ... 202
    1.5. Summary 207

Synthesis of the Chapter 208

General Evaluation and Conclusion 211

1. The Context of the Research 212
2. The Status of the Simple Case IVF-ET 213
3. Some Basic Points of Agreement between the Pros and Cons on the Simple Case 214
4. The Debate on the Simple Case Prior to *Donum Vitae* 214
5. The Debate after *Donum Vitae* 215
6. The Divergent Anthropologies and Approaches to the Simple Case 216

7. The Conjugal Act as the Most Fundamental Principle for the Rejection of the Simple Case 217

8. Other Principles against the Simple Case 217

9. Intentionality Is Not Sufficient in Itself to Justify the Use of the Simple Case 218

10. The Simple Case Offends against the Dignity of Human Procreation 219

Bibliography 223

Magisterium and other Statements from the Holy See 223

Primary Sources 224

    Works on the Simple Case 224

    Publications on *Donum Vitae* 226

Secondary Sources 232

    Theological Works on in Vitro Fertilization 232

General Theological Works 241

List of Abbreviations

AAS	*Acta Apostolicae Sedis*
Aa. Vv.	*Autori vari*, Various authors
AC	Artificial Conception
AF	Artificial Fertilization
AI	Artificial Insemination
AID	Artificial Insemination by Donor
AIH	Artificial Insemination by Husband
AP	Artificial Procreation
AR	Artificial Reproduction
ART	Artificial Reproductive Technology
ASS	*Acta Sanctae Sedis*
CDF	Congregation For the Doctrine of the Faith
Cf.	Confer (refer)
Ed./Eds.	Editor/Editors
Eng.	English
Et. al.	*Et alii* or *et alia*, And others
FIVET	*Fecondazione in vitro ed embryo transfer*
FIVETE	*Fécondation in vitro et Transfert d'embryons*
GIFT	Gamete IntraFallopian (tube) Transfer
GUIT	Gamete Intrauterine Transfer
Ibid.	*Ibidem* (in the same place)
ICSI	IntraCytoplasmic Sperm Injection
Introd.	Introduction
IVF-ET	In Vitro Fertilization and Embryo Transfer
LTOT	Low Tubal Ovum Transfer
MAP	Medical Assisted Procreation
n./nn.	Number/Numbers
TOTS	Tubal Ovum Transfer with Sperm
Trans.	Translation
Vol.	Volume

General Introduction

The gift of a child is a blessing from God and the fruit of conjugal union. Experience reveals that many couple desire to have a child in their marital union but this aspiration is not always realized in every marriage, perhaps due to certain pathological problems in the reproductive systems of either one or both of the spouses. Infertility in marriage can bring real pains and anxieties to any marriage. Hence the quest of couples to go all-out employing every possible medical means to overcome their condition is understandable, but deserves more importantly a moral guide. On 29 September 1949, Pius XII in his discourse to the Fourth International Congress of Catholic Physicians, condemned artificial insemination by husband (AIH) and in a similar discourse in 1956 extended the proscription to human in vitro fertilization that was then only a prediction. His action gave an indication to the wrongfulness and rejection of any form of intervention on human generation that separates procreation from the marital sexual act. The Pius XII's attention to the question of human artificial fertilization was a follow up to the response of 26 March 1897. At that time, the Holy Office, with the permission of Leo XIII, gave an emphatic NO answer without qualification to the question: "May artificial insemination of a woman be done?"[4] It seems theologians were not quite sure of the reason for the Vatican's negative response but presumed the involvement of the condition of masturbation to be the reason.[5] Up until the declaration made

---

4 Cf. *Response of the Holy Office*, 17 March 1897: in *ASS* 29 (26 March 1897): 704.
5 Cf. John C. Wakefield, *Artful Childmaking: Artificial Insemination in Catholic Teaching* (St. Louis, Missouri: The Pope John XXIII Medical-Moral Research and Education Center, 1978), 38. The study traces the history and theological developments regarding artificial insemination and reveals that the unqualified "no" response from the Congregation of the Inquisition in 1897, prompted different interpretations from moral theologians. It makes reference to an anonymous author who published a short article in the *Nouvelle Revue Theologique* shortly after the response of the Vatican on the matter and insinuated that artificial insemination even in marriage was condemned for reason that the sperm was obtained by means of masturbation. This article ignited two distinct interpretations to the magisterial response. The first opinion expressed in the

by Pius XII, artificial insemination by husband excluding masturbation was considered in theological discussions as an open question. Indeed, Pius XII was eloquent and consistent on this matter and repeated this teaching in 1951 and 1956 and in most of his discourses to relevant associations of medical professionals. He went further to assert that the condemnation of artificial insemination does not foreclose any means that could help couples in the performance of the conjugal act or assists the conjugal act normally performed to achieve its natural purpose. To this end, homologous artificial fertilization was in principle left open and the question on substitution and assistance to the conjugal act emerged. The Pope's intervention on the issue was impressive but could not resolve completely the controversy because another concern arose. The matter at stake was: what constitutes the nature of assistance or substitution as medical intervention on human procreation? Theologians would engage themselves in this debate for the next decades after Pius XII.

Twenty years after Pius XII's first declaration on the question of intervention on human procreation, the encyclical letter *Humanae Vitae* of Paul VI in 1968 argued strongly against the deliberate separation of the unitive and procreative meanings of the conjugal act based on sound reasoning and divine revelation taking into consideration the nature of the person and of his sexuality. While this argument was employed in that document to illustrate the intrinsically evil nature of contraception, the same principle properly applies to artificial insemination or artificial fertilization *in vitro*. By reason of seeking procreation outside the conjugal act, artificial insemination or in vitro fertilization is judged to be illicit. A decade after the release of *Humanae Vitae*, Louise Joy Brown was born at the Oldham district hospital in England as the first surviving so-called "Test Tube Baby" in history. Many people hailed this development as a triumph in biomedical

---

Journal cited above claims that artificial insemination was rejected because of immoral means used. Whereas, the second view published in the rival Journal, *Revue Theologique Francaise*, maintains in the contrary that any interference with the natural procreative process was illicit or immoral. The anonymous article was entitled, "foecundatio artificialis mulieris declaratur illicita," in *Nouvelle Revue Théologique* 29 (1897): 323-324. The second article is cited in Leon Renwart, "Insemination artificielle et documents pontificaux," in *Nouvelle Revue Théologique* 71 (1949): n8, 1073.

research. Since then, innumerable numbers of children are reported being born through IVF-ET. However, this procedure of human fertilization has remained a controversial subject and a matter of concern among moral theologians and religious bodies, individuals, biomedical professionals as well as governments. Varied responses have been expressed about this so-called groundbreaking achievement of the British team of Robert Edwards and Patrick Steptoe.

1. The Actual Problem

On 22 February 1987, the Congregation for the Doctrine of the Faith (CDF), having received information from various Episcopal Conferences, individual bishops, doctors and scientists on the joys, confusions, anxieties and uncertainties regarding the new reproductive technologies, published the *Instruction on Respect for Human Life in Its Origin and On the Dignity of Human Procreation* (*Donum Vitae*)[6] as a moral guide on the limits of interventions on human procreation. This Instruction proscribes as illicit procedures of artificial procreation that separate generation of human life from sexual intercourse including the so-called "Simple Case" IVF, i.e. a homologous IVF and ET procedure that is free of any compromise with the abortive practice of destroying embryos and with masturbation.[7] By rejecting even the simple case IVF procedure, *Donum Vitae* is generally seen as reaffirming the forceful assertion of Pius XII's teaching on the unity of the two aspects of the conjugal act; and specifically accepting the judgment of Paul VI in *Humanae Vitae*, that there is an unbreakable link between the marital sexual act and procreation willed by God the Creator

---

6 Congregation for the Doctrine of the Faith, *Instruction Donum Vitae, On Respect for Human Life in Its Origin and On the Dignity of Human Procreation*, 22 February 1987: in *AAS* 80 (1988): 70–102. English translation from Boston: Pauline Books and Media, 1987. The reference to this document will subsequently be: *Donum Vitae*.
7 Ibid., II, B/5. The "Simple Case" will hereafter be simply identified as either the simple case or the simple case IVF-ET. This procedure of in vitro fertilization is so called because it is adjudged to be clinically a simple procedure comparatively and morally less problematic because it is assumed to be free of abortive practices, embryos destruction and masturbation unlike the standard IVF.

which man cannot break on his own initiative. Some renowned Catholic theologians had thought that there would be exception to the simple case in the Church's negative judgment of some reproductive technologies since they considered it less problematic and limited to those in a marital union. However, the Instruction did not spare the simple case but judged it to be morally wrong for the primary reason, at least, of separating procreation from marital sexual intercourse thereby lacking the perfection belonging to human procreation by nature. In other words, the simple case by seeking to achieve procreation outside the specific sexual intercourse of couple, objectively effects an analogous separation between the goods and the meanings of marriage and equally of the unity in the conjugal act. The Church's judgment is informed by her conviction of the value of the intimate link between the unitive and procreative meanings of the sexual act based on the intrinsic unity of the human being as a bodily and spiritual creature. With this, the document reiterates the Church's teaching on the principle of inseparability of the conjugal act in its unitive and procreative dimensions, stressing that every marital sexual act requires openness to procreation and no procreation is to be initiated or sought outside the marital sexual act. In its conclusion the document calls upon moralists and theologians to reflect profoundly on relevant teachings of the Magisterium and apply this teaching to guide especially those involved in human procreation. Soon after the release of this document, a number of varied responses started featuring in different ways in scholarly Journals and Pastorals to the Instruction's invitation. Yet, important issues remained unresolved and required some clarifications and debates. Indeed, the teaching of *Donum Vitae* especially on the simple case IVF-ET evoked both affirmative and dissenting responses from within and outside the Catholic Church's theological circles. What can be said to be the main contention regarding the procedure in question and the opinions of Catholic moral theologians and ethicists?

2. The Main Argument

The problem of the simple case is theoretical but with practical implications which we shall indicate in the course of this study. Irrespective of the negative evaluation or rejection of the simple case by the Magisterium, some Catholic moralists known by Elio Sgreccia as "Possibilists" still believe that the simple case could be licit, thereby contending that the Instruction's conclusion is erroneous. The advocates of the simple case are concerned that the Instruction acknowledges the fact that the simple case as well as other forms of homologous IVF and ET procedures is not complicated by all that ethical negativity found in extra-conjugal procreation but it does not judge it worthy of human procreation. The basic reason given in the Instruction, which the dissenting theologians find inadequate is that it breaks the two intrinsically connected aspects of the conjugal act. Another problem is the ambiguity with which authors understand the simple case. While some authors talk of the simple case as a limited form of homologous IVF-ET and not yet in practice, still hypothetical, only possible in theory, others understand it in a broader perspective referring to any form of homologous IVF-ET performed in certain circumstances. This last part gives the impression that this procedure is already being performed. Generally, the clinical procedure of the simple case as described in theory is the same with that of standard IVF-ET currently in practice except in some aspects. Following the descriptions made by some scholars regarding the simple case IVF-ET, the general differences between this method and the standard IVF-ET could be found in the following aspects: (1) It does not involve masturbation; (2) Only limited embryos are fertilized and transferred; (3) It does not involve abortive practices; (4) The gametes are obtained in a "legitimate" way in the "context of marital love."[8] These are the basic clinical indications (in theory) of the simple case that differ from the standard IVF-ET. But, how simple is the so-called "simple case IVF-ET"? This poser underlines the basic arguments around this procedure.

---

8   Elio Sgreccia, *Personalistic Bioethics: Foundations and Applications*, Eng. Trans. John A. Di Camillo and Michael J. Miller (Philadelphia: The National Catholic Bioethics Center, 2012), 511. Expressing the views of the "Possibilists," Sgreccia notes that the means by which gametes are made available in homologous artificial insemination improperly speaking would be the same way in the simple case IVF-ET; the unity between the unitive and procreative dimensions of the conjugal act would be found in the "context of marital love" from which the request comes and in which conception occurs.

3. Objectives and Doctrinal Relevance of This Project

What will engage us in this research is to find out what can be derived from the diverse theological responses to the Instruction *Donum Vitae* by studying the literature and materials that have emerged in respect of the Instruction's conclusion on the simple case IVF-ET. In other words, this study is aimed at evaluating the moral-theological views of known Catholic authors on the problematic and hypothetic procedure of human generation – the simple case IVF-ET. In so doing, the moral tradition upon which each group of discussants is influenced by will be highlighted. Obviously, the work of this kind with relatively scarce bibliography and having the central problem of ambiguous terminological understandings among authors, poses extra challenges. The fact that this topic to our knowledge has not been treated or adequately discussed among Catholic theologians remains a strong stimulus for this project and indeed would make it more interesting and relevant. We need to state that before and after the instruction *Donum Vitae*, there has not been any monograph dedicated to this question of the simple case IVF-ET, at best there are only few articles.[9] Curiously, the only scholarly work dedicated almost entirely to this problem might probably be the *Journal of Philosophy and Medicine*, volume 53 published a decade after *Donum Vitae*. The publication authored by Thomas A. Shannon and Lisa Sowle Cahill, lay Catholic ethicists[10] is another response that is worthy of recognition.

---

9   Carol A. Tauer, "Dissenting Opinions on In Vitro Fertilization" in Kevin Wm. Wildes (ed.), *Infertility: A Crossroad of Faith, Medicine, and Technology* (Dordrecht/Boston/London: Kluwer Academic Publishers, 1997), 129. In this article, Tauer expresses the same view that there are little recent materials discussing the morality of the simple case. See also LeRoy Walters, Director of Kennedy Institute of Ethics who had described it as a "stagnant issue" far back in 1984 (cited by Richard A. McCormick, *The Critical Calling: Reflections on Moral Dilemma Since Vatican II* (Washington, D.C.: Georgetown University Press, 1989), 331. None of these authors offers useful reasons why the technique is rarely discussed; the only assumption would be that the Vatican has made a final pronouncement and may not change her position.
10 Thomas A. Shannon and Lisa Sowle Cahill, *Religion and Artificial Procreation: An Inquiry Into The Vatican "Instruction on Respect for Human Life"* (New York: Crossroad, 1988). The authors applaud the life-affirming aspects of the document, but also suggest that, under certain conditions, some

The earliest Catholic theologians who responded to the Instruction in various ways in support of the simple case IVF-ET would include Richard A. McCormick who describes the document as "unpersuasive" for condemning even the simple case.[11] Other renowned advocates of the simple case include, Lisa S. Cahill, Anthony Shannon, Patrick Vespieren, Edward Vacek, etc. They feel that the negative judgment on the simple case would place Catholic couples and medical professionals in a state of dilemma and frustration as they struggle with the challenge of infertility. It is reported that at least four Catholic Universities (Nimegen, Lille, and the two Louvains) expressed their views against the Instruction's judgment on the simple case and promised to continue providing in vitro fertilization for couples, this sounds like a protest! The chief administrator at Lille is said to have publicly doubted the moral evidence of illicity that he believes cannot be found in the document.[12] These theologians argue that the marital union should be the only context to evaluate the morality of artificial procreation and not every act of conjugal sexual love. For them, conjugal act should be understood in the perspective that it embraces the totality of the marital union and the activities performed for the sake of this union.

Furthermore, there are numerous monographs on the standard IVF-ET published before and after *Donum Vitae* from which allusions are made to the simple case. William E. May is probably one of the first Catholic theologians to publish an article specifically on the simple case IVF-ET in which he defends the magisterial judgment. There are other known authors like Elio Sgreccia, Nicholas Tonti-Filippini, Janet Smith, Germain Grisez, Ignacio Carrasco De Paula, John Boyle, Martin Rhonheimer, Josef Seifert, Ángel Rodríguez-Luño and many more who have expressed views that are

---

techniques like the simple case IVF-ET used between spouses may be morally acceptable.

11 Some works by McCormick that he expresses positive views on the simple case IVF-ET after the release of *Donum Vitae*: "Document is Unpersuasive," *In Responses to the Vatican Document on Reproductive Technologies* (St. Louis: The Catholic Health Association, 1987): 8–10; "The Vatican Document on Bioethics: Some Unsolicited Questions," in *America* 156 (1987): 24–28; "Begotten, not made," in *Notre Dame Magazine* (Autumn 1987): 22–25.

12 Cf. McCormick, *The Critical Calling*, 346.

supportive of *Donum Vitae's* position on the simple case as well, but not with specific works on this procedure.[13]

We find this work interesting and relevant because of our belief that the analysis of the arguments presented in this thesis will contribute to the understanding of the debate on the simple case and artificial procreation in general. The basic teaching of the Instruction on the simple case that we expound, will help readers to appreciate the doctrinal teaching position of the Church on the limits of intervention in human procreation. It is equally pertinent to remember that the Instruction *Donum Vitae* invites theologians and moralists for a deeper reflection on this problem and this research is no less a contribution in response to that call.

4. Methodology and Delimitation of the Work

The methodology of this thesis is expository, analytical and evaluative. Basic and general arguments employed by both those in support of the simple case and those in defense of the Instruction's judgment are presented with headings connected to the main themes of each section. The methodology is such that the magisterial doctrines and theological opinions in the first chapter will set in place the main work upon which the pros and cons arguments will be treated respectively. The advantage of placing in

---

13 Famous among the Catholic theologians who argue in defense of the Church's position are: William E. May, "The 'Simple Case' of In Vitro Fertilization and Embryo Transfer," in *Linacre Quarterly* 55,1 (1988): 29–36; Ibid., "*Donum Vitae*: Catholic Teaching Concerning Homologous In Vitro Fertilization," in *Philosophy and Medicine* 53 (1989): 73–92; Elio Sgreccia, "Moral Theology and Artificial Procreation in Light of *Donum Vitae*," in Edmund D. Pellegrino, John Collins Harvey and John P. Langan (eds.), *Gift of Life: Catholic Scholars Respond to the Vatican Instruction* (Washington, D.C: Georgetown University Press, 1990), 115–135; Joseph Boyle, "An Introduction to the Vatican Instruction on Reproductive Technologies," in *Linacre Quarterly* 55, 1 (1988): 20–28; Josef Seifert, "Substituting or Replacing the Conjugal Act or Assistance to It? IVF, GIFT and Some other Medical Interventions, Philosophical Reflections on the Vatican Declaration *Donum Vitae*," in *Anthropotes* 4 (1988): 273–286 and Ángel Rodríguez-Luño, "The Continuity of the Magisterial Teaching," in United States Conference of Catholic Bishops (ed.), *Instruction Donum Vitae: Commentaries and Studies* (Washington, D.C.: Libreria Editrice Vaticana, 2013): 38–44.

the second chapter the arguments of the dissenting theologians will help us to feel the impulse and weight of their critiques against the magisterial teaching in *Donum Vitae* and respond adequately with the defending theological views favorable to the Instruction in the third chapter. In so doing, the work will clarify the teaching of the Magisterium as well as respond to criticisms arising from the dissenting theological views. Each of the chapters will have a synthesis. Since there are scarce specific articles on the simple case, perhaps because the problem is still evolving, the work will make some inferences and assumptions from general discussions on the standard IVF-ET and similar procedures since the simple case is a (theoretical) species of IVF-ET. Since the simple case is a theoretical procedure, the work is not focused on the clinical indications of this method but limited to the moral and theological debate within the Catholic circle. This implies that we shall not delve into the laboratory process of this technique but we will however give a brief description of its aspects in a footnote. We are aware of the legal, social and economic perspectives of the debate on this problem within and outside the Catholic Church, but our focus principally is on its moral and theological aspect.

While the work makes use of literature from Italian, German, Spanish, French and English languages, it is predominated by bibliography in English language. The simple reason is that the research is undertaken in English that is more convenient and expedient for the researcher. Our study spans from the period of *Casti Connubii* to *Donum Vitae* and extends to the present time. It is pertinent to indicate that one of the major challenges of this work is the lack of precise and specific bibliography on the simple case. In addition, we made efforts to investigate in the Vatican archives the claim made by the dissenting theologians on inadequate or selective consultations in the drafting of the Instruction *Donum Vitae* but it was not successful owing to the reason that such documents are not open to the public within few years. It was aimed to evaluate how extensive the consultation was whether considerable consultations were made as mentioned by Joseph Cardinal Ratzinger or the opposite as held by critics of the document.[14]

---

14 Joseph Ratzinger made this claim during the Vatican Press Conference of 10 March 1987 was published in *L'Osservatore Romano*, English edition (16 March 1987), 8.

However, it is unlikely that the validity of arguments on the morality of the simple case IVF-ET is dependent on consultations or similar matters but on the nature of the procedure itself.

5. Organization of Chapters

The work is structured in three chapters enclosed by the general introduction and conclusion. The introductory section gives a general direction of problem, purpose methodology, structure and arguments of the thesis.

In Chapter One we will give a synthetic presentation of some magisterial teachings dealing with the principles that relate to human procreation and means of generating human life. The goal is to investigate the foundation and development of the Catholic moral doctrines and theological opinions that could apply to the simple case IVF-ET. There are two major sections of this chapter: the first section is dealing with the papal teachings as well as theological opinions of some Catholics. This section constitutes arguments that pertain to the simple case prior to *Donum Vitae*. In the second section however, an overview of the Instruction *Donum Vitae* is treated with particular interest on issues that concern the simple case. The three lines of reasoning as the main arguments of the document on artificial procreation are expounded.

Experience reveals that there are always some reactions to the Church's official declarations. And so, the Chapter Two of this work covers the dissenting theological opinions on the simple case in the light of the Instruction's judgment. This chapter explores critically the opinions of the dissenting theologians on the simple case as a possible method to assist infertile couples to achieve procreation in their marital union. The chapter under consideration is divided into three main sections treating the principal arguments considered by the dissenters to constitute the inadequacy of the Instruction's judgment as well as their support for the simple case. In the first section, the critiques of the document are presented, contending that the document is deficient in its methodology and profusely characterized by assumptions. In the second section, it focuses on the conjugal act and the claim of the error of reductionism of the Instruction. In other words, the dissenting theologians claim that the conjugal act is not limited or should not be reduced to the sexual act of the couple as we are made to believe, but extended to the totality of conjugal life. And so, the simple case could be licit to assist the couple to have children in some circumstances because it can be an extension of the conjugal act. In the third section, the dissenting theological opinion claims that the child is begotten and not made in the simple case contrary to the teaching implied in *Donum Vitae* and spoken of by some theologians. Hence, the moral object of the simple case is misunderstood in the document and by its defenders; the moral object of the procedure would be in the intention of the couples and not in the procedure itself as implied in the document.

In response to the critiques of the dissenting views and in support of *Donum Vitae*'s judgment on the simple case, Chapter Three articulates the argument of those in sympathy with the document and opposed to the simple case procedure. This chapter is divided into three sections with specific themes related to the basic principles that are used to evaluate the simple case. The first section expounds on the anthropological and theological foundation of the Instruction's argument to refute the claim by the dissenting opinion that the document's anthropology and methodology lack integral vision of the human person. In the second section, the argument revolves around the dignity of human procreation underscoring the uniqueness and profundity of the conjugal act as the morally licit source of human procreation. This section is emphatic that the conjugal act is a personal act, irreplaceable by any other action and cannot be performed on someone's behalf. Following this conclusion, it contends that the simple case is a replaceable act and by that fact a non-marital act and so unworthy of being the origin of the child. The third section takes up the argument against the simple case based on the teaching that the child is "begotten, not made." This section argues that the simple case replaces the conjugal act and does not assist it as claimed by its proponents. It also emphasizes that the desire of couples to have a child or actual result of fertilization cannot justify the use of the simple case because the procedure is intrinsically disordered in its moral object and implies that the child is *something* to be produced and not *someone* to be begotten.

Chapter One The Magisterium and Some Theological Opinions on Artificial Procreation

Introduction

Artificial intervention on human procreation has been a problematic topic in legal, moral and bioethical debates. The birth of Louise Joy Brown on 25 July 1978 by means of in vitro fertilization and embryo transfer (IVF-ET)[15] procedure is the most significant event that marks the "high point" in medical assisted procreation that was merely a theoretical problem in

---

15 The Technology of IVF-ET is a combination of two separate procedures that are usually involved when procreation is sought by means of extra-corporal fertilization. The IVF that is performed in view of procreation will need the embryos to be transferred to the woman's body. This suggests that it is not every IVF that involves embryo transfer. IVF is the first major procedure preceded by other series of events. For example, in most cases, the woman's ovaries are stimulated with fertility drugs to produce multiple eggs monitored by the physician. Subsequently, the ova of the woman are harvested by means of laparoscope from the ovary shortly before it would have been released naturally. The ova can also be collected by means of transvaginal aspiration, done with local anaesthesia; the physician inserts the needle through the woman's vagina, guided by ultrasound. What follows is the mixture of the ova with the sperm (the semen previously collected either by masturbation or collected during sexual intercourse using condom) in a medium, so that fertilization can occur externally in a test tube. Fertilization of the egg occurs approximately over the period of twelve to eighteen hours in the incubator. The temperature and condition of this medium are designed to mimic that of the human body. After about forty-eight to seventy hours, the fertilized egg would have started dividing into two or more cells. And then, they are placed in a catheter, a hollow needle and inserted into the woman's vagina and the embryos are released into the uterus for onward possible development. This last procedure is called embryo transfer (ET). Cf. Andrea L. Bonnicksen, "Reproductive Technologies: In Vitro Fertilization and Embryo Transfer," in Warren T. Reich (ed.), *Encyclopedia of Bioethics*, Vol. 4 (New York: The Free Press, 1995), 2221. Hereafter in this work, we shall refer to this procedure as in vitro fertilization and embryo transfer or by its acronym – IVF-ET.

the Mid 20th Century.[16] The "success" of this medical effort was a result of long advances and experiments in infertility treatment that began with experimentations on animals and eventually human artificial insemination.[17] Advances in ART were attended by ethical, legal, religious and social concerns and various governments and groups have always made attempts to regulate the use of these technologies in human procreation.

---

16 The concepts: "Medical Assisted Procreation" (MAP), "Artificial Reproductive Technology" (ART), "Assisted Reproductive Technology" (ART), "Artificial Procreation" (AP), "Artificial Reproduction" (AR), "Artificial Conception" (AC) and "Artificial Fertilization" (AF), etc., have been used by authors differently but largely referring to the same reality. Generally, authors use any of them to refer to the use of a medical technique or procedure to achieve human fertilization. Among authors who use these concepts, many use them without bothering about their ethical or moral significance. However, some make attempt to indicate that using the terms such as "reproduction" to refer to the generation of human life would be improper because man procreates and not only "reproduce." For such authors, reproduction implies re-producing which is morally wrong in the light of human dignity. Rather, procreation is considered to be the right term because it signifies co-creating with God, in this way it becomes clear that human life is begotten and not reproduced like in lower animals. Some also think that the use of the term "assisted procreation" by some authors to refer to a human extra-corporal fertilization is misleading, because what is involved in laboratory fertilization is not truly assistance or aid to the conjugal act but substitution through mechanical manipulations of the procreative process. However, in this work, the terms will be used most times liberally in the biological sense to refer to medical intervention in human procreation. In our evaluation we shall take into consideration the moral relevance of these concepts and thereby indicate the proper concepts that can be appropriate to be used in referring to medical assistance in human procreation.
17 Cf. Robert Edwards and Patrick Steptoe, *A Matter of Life: The Story of a Medical Breakthrough* (New York: William Morrow and Company, Inc., 1980); Elio Sgreccia, *Personalist Bioethics*, 495–539; Andrea L. Bonnicksen, *In Vitro Fertilization: Building Policy from Laboratories to Legislatures* (New York: Columbia University Press, 1989), 11–24; James A. Simon, "Advances in Assisted Reproductive Technologies," in *Philosophy and Medicine* 53 (1997): 53–71; Lawrence J. Kaplan and Carolyn M. Kaplan, "Natural Reproduction and Reproduction-Aiding Technologies," in Kenneth D. Alpern (ed.), *The Ethics of Reproductive Technology* (New York: Oxford University Press, 1992), 15–31.

The Warnock report[18] is one of such attempts by the British government and it has been widely accepted to be influential in the policies of other governments regarding artificial procreation. The committee recommended a number of techniques such as AID, IVF, egg and embryo donation, the clinical use of frozen embryos. It equally proposed the use of embryos for research up to the fourteenth day under licensing. However, the Warnock report disapproved of the use of embryo donation by lavage, surrogacy and cloning, etc. On the recommendation of the use of embryos for research, one group of dissents argued: "although, 'it is right that efforts should be made to alleviate' infertility, and although 'the advance of scientific knowledge is likewise of great value', neither of these ends justifies the 'deliberate destruction' of human embryos."[19]

Before the Warnock Committee was inaugurated, the Catholic Church as an institution that is said to be "an expert in humanity" with the mission to serve the "civilization of love" and the custodian of human life had responded at different times to the question of artificial intervention in human procreation. The impact of the magisterial response to this most basic aspect of humanity, that is, human procreation cannot be overemphasized. This first chapter of our study treats the magisterial interventions and some

---

18 This is the report of the British committee of inquiry established in July 1982 headed by Dame Mary Helen Warnock, to examine the social, ethical and legal implications of developments in the field of human assisted fertilization. This report was submitted on 26 June 1984. It is commonly called the Warnock report. See Mary Warnock, *A Question of Life: Report of the Committee of Inquiry into Human Fertilization and Embryology* (Oxford: Blackwell Publishers, 1993), 4.

19 Ibid, 90–93. See also Nigel M. de S. Cameron, "The Christian Take in the Warnock Debate," in Nigel M. de S. Cameron (ed.), *Embryos and Ethics: The Warnock Report in Debate* (Edinburg: Rutherford House Books, 1987), 2–3. Cameron alleges that there was a bias in setting the committee, indicating that persons of pronounced opinion were not considered and are not generally considered for committees of inquiry, which are designed to provide compromises. He feels that in the said committee, none of the moral philosophers or Churchmen with conservative positions on ethical issues was invited for the discussion. He claims those who even dissented still lacked the knowledge of the true status of the embryo because they argued on the ground of "potential" and not "actual" personhood of the embryo. This negative situation raises suspicion on the validity of the committee and of the report.

theological responses on the problem of artificial procreation from *Casti Connubii* to *Donum Vitae*.

A. Magisterial Teachings on Artificial Procreation Prior to *Donum Vitae*

The first time the problem of artificial fertilization appeared under moral evaluation in official Church documents was in the answer from the Sacred Congregation of the Universal Inquisition now known as the Congregation for the Doctrine of the Faith, on 14 March 1897. The question was framed: "May Artificial Insemination be applied to a woman?" And the precise response was: "No."[20] The question was borne out of the controversy generated at the time among theologians on the licitness or illicitness of artificial insemination. This response that had no further explanation or substantiation yet entered in the *Code of Cannon Law* of 1917 repudiating artificial insemination explicitly.[21] In the following discussion, we will undertake an investigation on subsequent magisterial response and elaboration on the subject, which in the preceding years was not given a profound justification to the answer given by the Vatican in 1897.

1.1. The Teaching of Pius XI: *Casti Connubii*, 31 December 1930

Pope Pius XI's Pontificate spanned from 1922 to 1939. He presided over the Church at the time the institution of marriage was being besieged by some

---

20 Cf. *Response of the Holy Office*: in *ASS* 29 (26 March 1897): 704. In Latin the question asked was: "*An adhiberi posit artificialis mulieris fecundatio?*" and the response from the Holy Office approved by Leo XIII was an emphatic: "*Non Licere*."

21 The 1917 *Code of Canon Law*, Can. 1068. § 3. "Sterilitas matrimonium nec dirimit nec impedit." (Sterility neither invalidates marriage nor renders it illicit). It is likely that this canon was aimed at settling the crisis in marriage caused by sterility that might have caused couples to resort to artificial insemination. It can be recalled that procreation was for long taught to be the primary end of marriage; and so the problem of childless marriage was understandably unbearable leaving couples with no option but to choose artificial insemination. This canon seems to address the fact that sterility cannot render a valid marriage invalid in light of the response of the Holy Office that artificial insemination was illicit.

negative forces and errors including the civil legislative policies derived from the negative humanism of that century. The civil governments of the day relaxed the laws on divorce and the resultant effects, one would say, included sexual revolution and disregard for the institution of marriage. Some people who held secular ideas thought of marriage as an institution that is purely of human origin and so should be divorced of religious association and regulations. Connected with this reality were the biomedical developments of contraceptive and reproductive technologies. The Pope's desire was to restore the institution of marriage to its proper dignity as intended by God, the institutor of matrimony. The response of Pius XI to this challenge was the encyclical On Christian Marriage *Casti Connubii*.[22]

This document did not address specifically the problem of artificial procreation rather it discussed the nature and dignity of Christian marriage. But, the discussion on marriage would obviously and necessarily include the question of procreation. It is in the light of this fact that the document touches the theme of our study – artificial procreation. True to this, the document indicates that the gift of children (procreation) is one of the blessings of holy matrimony which couples have the "power and right to beget."[23] It is relevant to note that Pius XI issued this document some months following the Church of England's declaration of support for contraception at Lambeth which the society found delight with.[24] At the time, contraception was commonplace and constituted almost the predominant public moral debate. Hence, one of the central objectives of this document was the condemnation of all forms of contraception. Since both contraception and artificial reproduction entail a separation of the two aspects of the conjugal act, the principles of this document can be directly or indirectly

---

22 Pius XI, Encyclical *Casti Connubii*, 31 December 1930: in *AAS* 22 (1930): 546–547.
23 *Casti Connubii*, n. 16. The implication of this statement is to point out that civil laws should not contravene or be made contrary to what God, the author of marriage has inscribed in the couples by virtue of their marital union.
24 At this famous *Lambeth Conference of Anglican Church* held on 15 August 1930, they voted for contraception with the vote aggregates: 193 in favor; 67 against and 47 abstained. As one of the mainline Christian bodies, its approval of contraception obviously signaled danger for the institution of marriage and attendant effects such as sexual indiscipline in the society.

applied to both problems but on different levels. For instance, it is contained in this document, although not very clearly, the principle of inseparability of the unitive and procreative significance of the conjugal act. The document indicates that: "...the conjugal act is destined primarily by nature for the begetting of children, those who in exercising it deliberately frustrate its natural power and purpose sin against nature and commit a deed which is shameful and intrinsically vicious."[25] No doubt, the above citation speaks clearly against contraception and was intended so, but it gives an insight to be applied to the act of frustrating the natural context from which the power of generating human life comes from, namely the sexual intercourse. In another section, it states, "every sin committed as regards the offspring becomes in some way a sin against conjugal faith, since both these blessings are *essentially connected*."[26]

Furthermore, this document contains some principles that could be applied to the problem of artificial procreation notwithstanding the fact that the document's specific intention was not artificial conception but contraception on account of the nature and dignity of marriage as a divine institution for communion and procreation. Pius XI indicates that matrimony is an institution ordained by God, the author of marriage and restored by our Lord Jesus Christ making it a sacrament. This affirmation of the nature of matrimony reveals it to be a sacred and noble institution to be preserved in all its dimensions. It is within this context that the gift of life from God is to be received. Highlighted in the document is the truth that matrimony is characterized by indissolubility and conjugal fidelity.[27]

Based on the nature of the human person and the moral teaching of the Church derived from natural law and Christian revelation, the emphasis laid on the blessings of marriage as children and conjugal fidelity become clear. The truth that is central to the document is that marriage is the only proper context for procreation and it depends not solely on man's will but the law of God. It affirms that "the duty entrusted to parents for the good of their children is of such high dignity and of such great importance, every use of the faculty given by God for the procreation of new life is the right and

---

25 *Casti Connubii*, n. 54.
26 Ibid., n. 72. (The emphasis is added).
27 Ibid., nn. 19 and 32.

the privilege of the married state alone, by the law of God and of nature, and must be confined absolutely within the sacred limits of that state."[28]

The teaching of this document does not immediately argue to support the response of Leo XIII against the application of artificial insemination on a woman. However, the principles of the document somehow laid the foundation that Pius XII would develop against some procedures of artificial procreation. In fact, *Casti Connubii* reiterates the Church's teaching that, marriage is a sacred bond of privilege and responsibility. Safeguarding the dignity of the conjugal act even in the challenge of infertility is an expression of that responsibility which marriage requires from spouses.

1.2. The Teaching of Pius XII

Pius XII led the Church on the throne of St. Peter the apostle from 2 March 1939 up until 9 October 1958. Pius XII's papacy coincided with the Second World War and an historic era of global political unrest and abuses against the family life. While the Pope did not write any encyclical letter specifically on marriage or sexual morality, he did give many speeches and messages on such issues as marriage, sexual morality, medicine and particularly on the limits of medical intervention in human procreation. In his teaching, he reaffirms and highlights most of the magisterial teachings of the previous Popes. For instance, he affirms that procreation is the primary purpose of marriage, the view his immediate predecessor had taught. Equally, Pius XII continues with the doctrine on the principle of the unity of the conjugal act in its unitive and procreative meanings, the principle stated in *Casti Connubii*. Pius XII employed this principle in his teaching against artificial insemination, a practice that was becoming a common infertility treatment in medicine at the time. He is considered the Pope who first started elaborating on the question of artificial procreation, the problem that was first attended to seminally by the Holy Office in 1897. Pius XII delivered several speeches to scientists, medical professionals and researchers. He

---

28 Ibid., n. 18. "...cum tantae dignitatis tantique momenti sit utrumque hoc munus parentibus in bonum prolis commissum, facultatis a Deo ad novam vitam procreandam datae honestus quilibet usus, ipso Creatore ipsaque naturae lege iubentibus, solius matrimonii ius est àc privilegium et intra sacros connubii limites est omnino continendus."

frequently addressed doctors, nurses and midwives, instructing them on the moral responsibilities of their professions and the right and dignity of patients and of marriage.

Similarly, this work will not concern the teachings of Pius XII in general but attention will be paid specifically to his teaching regarding medical intervention on human procreation. The Pope's orientation regarding the nascent human life and the sanctity of marriage depended on the ontological moral tradition, relying heavily on the natural law and personalist morality.

1.2.1. Address to the International Congress of Catholic Medical Doctors, 29 September 1949

The Pope's address to the Catholic Medical Doctors on the occasion of their Fourth International Congress[29] comprising thirty nations held in Rome on Thursday, 29 September 1949, was the first of its kind to address more elaborately the Church's objection to artificial insemination. This speech is considered by many as an epoch making event inasmuch as the moral debate on artificial procreation is concerned. In view of the progress in medicine and the moral responsibilities of doctors in the practice of their noble profession in the service of life, the Pope underscores four main principles in objection to artificial insemination. From the point of view of Catholic moral tradition, Pius XII's objection to artificial insemination as he indicates, would be a bit broad and derived from the moral judgment that governs it. According to him:

1. When dealing with humans, the question of artificial insemination cannot be considered neither exclusively – nor yet principally – under its biological and medical aspect, leaving aside the moral and juridical point of view.

---

29 Pius XII, *Discourse to the Fourth International Congress of Catholic Doctors*, 29 September 1949: in *AAS* 41 (1949): 557–561. This document will be cited in this as: *Discourse to the Fourth International Congress of Catholic Doctors*. The special audience took place at the Papal residence in Castel Gandolfo. The text of the message was in French language but the English translation source is from: Peter Hünermann (ed.), *Heinrich Denzinger, Compendium of Creeds, Definitions, and Declarations on Matters of Faith and Morals*: 3873a, 43rd Edition (San Francisco: Ignatius Press, 2012), 798–799.

2. Artificial insemination outside marriage must be condemned as immoral purely and simply. In fact the natural law and divine positive law state that the procreation of new life cannot take place except in marriage. Only marriage safeguards the dignity of the partners – in the present case principally that of the woman- their personal wellbeing, and guarantees at the same time the wellbeing of the child and his upbringing. It follows that there cannot be any difference of opinion among Catholics regarding the condemnation of artificial insemination outside the conjugal union. The child born under these conditions would be by that very fact illegitimate.
3. Artificial insemination in matrimony, but produced by means of the active element of a third person, is equally immoral, and as such is to be condemned without right of appeal. Only the husband and wife have the reciprocal right on the body of the other for the purpose of generating new life: an exclusive, inalienable, incommunicable right. And that is as it should be, also for the sake of the child. To whoever gives life to any creature, nature imposes, in virtue of that very bond, the duty of protecting and educating the child. But when the child is the fruit of the active elements of a third person-even granting the husband's consent- between the legitimate husband and the child there is no such bond of origin, nor the normal and juridical bond of conjugal procreation.
4. What of the liceity of artificial insemination in matrimony? For the moment let it suffice to recall the principles of the natural law: the mere fact that the means reaches the goal intended does not justify the use of such a means. Nor the desire for a child, a completely legitimate desire of the couples, suffices to prove that recourse to artificial fecundation is legitimate because it would satisfy such a desire.[30]

The Pope equally indicated that it would be wrong to reason that artificial insemination in a marriage between persons who are incapable of contracting it by the fact of impediment of impotence (*impedimentum*

---

30 Ibid. "Quant à licéité de la fécondation artificielle dans le mariage, qu'il Nous suffise, pour l'instant, de rappeler ces principes de droit naturel: le simple fait que le résultat auquel on vise est atteint par cette voie, ne justifie pas l'emploi du moyen lui-même; ni le désir, en soi très légitime chez les époux, d'avoir un enfant, nè sufiit à prouver la légitimité du recours à la fécondation artificielle, qui réaliserait ce désir," 560

impotentiae) could validate such a union. He also gives an indication of condemnation about masturbation when he states that: "... it goes without saying that the active element (gamete) can never be procured licitly by acts that are contrary to nature."[31]

However, Pius XII having outlined these conditions goes on to state that it is not every method of artificial procreation that is considered illicit. This indicates that certain techniques designed solely to assist the conjugal act to achieve its natural purpose could be morally acceptable. He substantiates that:

> Though new methods cannot be excluded a priori simply because they are new, in the case of artificial insemination one should not only keep a very cautious reserve, but must exclude it altogether. This does not necessarily forbid the use of certain artificial means destined simply either to facilitate the natural act, or to enable the natural act, normally carried out, to attain its proper end.[32]

Furthermore, he sustains that only the procreation of a new life according to the will and the plan of the Creator carries with it, to an amazing degree of perfection, the realization of intended aims. It is at the same time, in conformity with the corporal and spiritual nature and dignity of the marriage partners, and with the normal and happy development of the child. These principles enumerated by Pius XII would later become the foundation for moral deliberations on artificial fertilization and infertility treatments. In essence, Pius XII condemns all the techniques of artificial procreation that undermine or actively substitute for the conjugal act. Curiously, while he says of artificial insemination outside of marriage and in the case of donor (AID) as being "immoral," he simply uses the term "must be entirely rejected" for the one in marriage using the husband's gamete (AIH). In any case, this does not imply that he considers this one to be right, rather, it could mean that it is less complicated and not morally wrong like others.

---

31 Ibid. "... il est superflu d'observer que l'élément actif ne peut jamais être procuré licitement par des actes contre nature."
32 Ibid. "Bien que l'on ne puisse *a priori* exclure de nouvelles méthodes, pour le seul motif de leur nouveauté, néanmoins, en ce qui touche la fécondation artificielle, non seulement il y a lieu d'être extrêmement réservé, mais il faut absolument l'écarter. En parlant ainsi, on ne proscrit pas nécessairement l'emploi de certains moyens artificiels destinés uniquement soit à faciliter l'acte naturel, soit à faire atteindre sa fin à l'acte naturel normalement accompli."

However, he encourages that those means that can simply assist the conjugal act to achieve its natural goal of begetting a child may be utilized.

1.2.2. Allocution to the Italian Catholic Union of Midwives, 29 October 1951

In this document, Pius XII expounds on man's collaborative vocation with nature to realize God's will and plan: "When one thinks of this admirable collaboration of the parents, of nature and of God, from which is born a new human being in the image and likeness of God, how can the precious contribution which you give to such a work be not appreciated?"[33] In this address he reminds the midwives of the responsibilities which their profession imposes on them. The Pope touches on a number of issues that relate to what he indicates as "professional apostolate of midwives" in his discourse, but this study will limit itself to the aspect on the ethics of medical intervention in human procreation, the aspect that concerns this study.

The Pope without outlining the principles already indicated in his previous address to the Catholic medical doctors in 1949, nevertheless, applies such principles in his discourse to the midwives. He sustains that God is the Creator of human life, and man as the creature of the Creator has natural limits in his collaboration with God to bring about a new human life. On the order which nature has set regarding the origin of life, the Pope indicates that:

> ... he who approaches this cradle of life's origin and exercises his action in one way or another must know the order which the Creator wishes to be maintained and the laws which govern it. For here it is not a case of purely physical or biological laws which blind forces and irrational agents obey, but of laws whose execution and effects are entrusted to the voluntary and free cooperation of man. This order, fixed by the supreme intelligence, is directed to the purpose willed by the Creator. It embraces the exterior work of man and the internal assent of his free will; it implies action and dutiful omission. Nature places at man's disposal

---

33 Pius XII, *Allocution to the Union of Italian Catholic Midwives*, 29 October 1951: in *AAS* 43 (1951): 835–854. This document will hereafter be cited as: *Allocution to the Union of Italian Catholic Midwives*. Allocution is described as a formal speech, especially one of incontrovertible or hortatory nature. As it patterns to the Church, it refers to a pronouncement delivered by the Pope to a targeted group, especially on a matter of policy or of great relevance.

the concatenation of the causes from which will raise a new human life, it is for man to release its loving force, for nature to develop its course and lead it to its completion. When man has completed his part and placed in action the marvelous evolution of life, his duty is to respect its progress in a religious manner, a duty which forbids him to arrest nature's work or halt its natural development.[34]

The Pope recalls here the two main forces that can work against the origin of human life – contraception and artificial fertilization. These two principles attack obviously the cradle of human life as they break the intrinsic unity between love union and procreation of the conjugal act.

In highlighting the first line of his teaching against artificial insemination, Pius XII notes, "to reduce the common life of husband and wife and the conjugal act to a mere organic function for the transmission of seed would be but to convert the domestic hearth, the family sanctuary, into a biological laboratory."[35] The Pope explains further and more specifically on the conjugal act saying:

> The conjugal act, in its natural structure, is a personal action, a simultaneous and immediate cooperation of husband and wife, which by the very nature of the agents and the propriety of the act, is the expression of the reciprocal gift, which, according to Holy Writ, effects the union 'in one flesh'. That is much more than the union of two genes, which can be effected even by artificial means, that is, without the natural action of husband and wife. The conjugal act, ordained and desired by nature, is a personal cooperation, to which husband and wife, when contracting marriage, exchange the right.[36]

Pius XII expresses in this discourse his personalist moral view, paying attention to the person and his action to be at the center for moral judgment on this matter. He is convinced that the conjugal act is the most personal and

---

34 Ibid.
35 Ibid., *Address to the Fourth International Congress of Italian Medical Doctors.*
36 Ibid., *Allocution to the Union of Italian Catholic Midwives*, 850. "L'atto coniugale, nella sua struttura naturale, è un'azione personale, una cooperazione simultanea e immediata dei coniugi, la quale, per la stessa natura degli agenti e la proprietà dell'atto, è la espressione del dono reciproco, che, secondo la parola della Scrittura, effettua l'unione (in una carne sola). Ciò è molto più della unione di due germi, la quale si può effettuare anche artificialmente, vale a dire senza l'azione naturale dei coniugi. L'atto coniugale, ordinato e voluto dalla natura, è una cooperazione personale, alla quale gli sposi, nel contrarre il matrimonio, si scambiano il diritto."

non-delegable act; a human act that is most sacred to the spouses themselves and if this is deliberately disregarded or relinquished in procreation, then the whole activity becomes morally wrong. His argument would also be against masturbation and gamete donation as he indicates in his discourse of 1949, because these acts were common and associated with artificial insemination at the period.[37] In general, the Pius XII in this second address places emphasis on the personal values of the marital act as well as the primary and secondary ends of marriage.

1.2.3. *Allocution to Participants at the Second World Congress on Infertility and Sterility, 19 May 1956*

The Pope's return to the discussion on artificial procreation in his Allocution to Participants of the Second World Congress on Infertility and Sterility is indicative of the seriousness of this problem. He had to give a sound moral direction on the matter owing to the all-round challenges of ethical, legal and social dimensions that the new techniques of human procreation were posing. The Pope was insistent that the means to assist human procreation in the case of infertility must not replace or endanger the conjugal act as the source of new human life and binding force in marital life. In the light

---

37 Cf. John C. Wakefield, *Artful Childmaking: Artificial Insemination in Catholic Teaching* (St. Louis, Missouri: Pope John XXIII Medical-Moral Research and Education Centre, 1978), 45. Wakefield insinuates that in the Mid 20th Century donor insemination as a therapy was growing rapidly which attracted some theological discussions and magisterial decisions. As regard masturbation, see *Discourse to the Fourth International Congress of Catholic Doctors*. Here, among other things Pius XII talks about procuring the active element by illicit acts that are contrary to nature. One understands this active element to be the gamete necessary for fertilization and the illicit act to be an act of masturbation by which means the gamete is made available for insemination. Furthermore, some authors like Martin Richards has confirmed that donor insemination was becoming a common clinical practice in the 1930s: "By the 1930s AID was being more widely used clinically in Britain (and elsewhere) as a medical solution to male infertility for married couples." See Martin Richards, "Artificial Insemination and Eugenics: Celibate Motherhood, Eutelegenesis and Germinal Choice," in *Studies in History and Philosophy of Science Part C: Studies in History and Philosophy of Biological and Biomedical Sciences* 39, 2 (2008): 211–221, at 221.

of this, Pius XII repeats the magisterial repudiation of artificial insemination and in addition mentions explicitly for the first time artificial human fecundation *in vitro* as methods of artificial procreation that separate procreation from the unitive dimension of marital life.[38]

In reiterating the Church's opposition to the two attitudes of either seeking procreation without bodily relation (artificial procreation) and bodily satisfaction without generation of new life (artificial contraception), the Pope argues for the inseparability of the unity of the two meanings of the conjugal act. He emphasizes that the spouses must not become egoistic by seeking emotional and physical gratification for themselves alone at the expense of begetting children out of their bodily union.[39] The Pope considers the deliberate avoidance of children in marriage as an act of selfishness. In this address, he calls attention to the opposite tendency of desiring a child outside of bodily union:

> But the Church has likewise ruled out the opposite attitude that purports to separate in generation, the biological activity in the personal relationship of

---

38 In his discourses, Pius XII did not seem to give the definitions of either AI or IVF. It may be helpful to observe the difference between these two methods of artificial procreation noted in the Pope's discussions. Artificial insemination is different from in vitro fertilization. Artificial insemination involves the deposition of the sperm into the woman's uterus by means of a syringe or similar means during ovulation so as to fertilize the egg. Fertilization occurs inside the body of the woman but not as the result of a conjugal act. The sperm can come from either the woman's husband or from a donor. This procedure was originally developed for use in animal husbandry to increase farm yields but was later used as infertility treatment for childless couples. On the other hand, in vitro fertilization (IVF) involves and entails the retrieval of the preovulatory ovum from the woman's ovary followed by a mixture with the sperm for fertilization to occur in a culture dish and subsequent development of the *conceptus* to the 2 to 8 cell stage. In other words, human IVF means the fertilization of the human egg outside the human body in a test tube unlike artificial insemination that fertilization occurs inside the body of the woman. Both procedures are achieved not as the result of the conjugal sexual act.

39 Cf. Pius XII, *Allocution to Participants of the Second World Congress on Infertility and Sterility*, 19 May 1956: in *AAS* 48 (1956): 465–474. The original text was in French but the translation is done by the researcher. Hereafter this document will be cited as: *Allocution to Participants of the Second World Congress on Infertility and Sterility*.

the spouses. The child is the fruit of the conjugal union, the fullness of which contributes to the organic functions, and sensitive emotions that bring into play the spiritual and selfless love of the soul. It is in the unity of this human act that we should consider the biological conditions of generation. Never is it permitted to separate these various aspects to the positive exclusion either of the procreative intention or the conjugal relationship. The relationship that unites the father and mother to the child has its root in the organic act and even more so in the deliberate gesture of the spouses and the willingness to mutually donate themselves to each other that finds its true fulfilment in the being that they put in the world.[40]

Furthermore, the Pope mentions particularly the foreseen method of artificial fertilization *in vitro* that he requests that it would be sufficient to reject it as immoral and absolutely illicit. He observes: "regarding the experiments in artificial insemination "in vitro," let it be sufficient to observe that they be rejected as immoral and absolutely illicit."[41]

Pius XII would have to give this directive against those methods of human artificial procreation to professional bodies whose jobs are directly related to medical practice because after his first speech on the problem, controversies dealing with approval and disapproval ensued among theologians.

---

[40] "Mais l'Eglise a écarté aussi l'attitude opposée qui prétendrait séparer, dans la génération, l'activité biologique de la relation personnelle des conjoints. L'enfant est le fruit de l'union conjugale, lorsqu'elle s'exprime en plénitude, par la mise en œuvre des fonctions organiques, des émotions sensibles qui y sont liées, de l'amour spirituel et désintéressé qui l'anime; c'est dans l'unité de cet acte humain que doivent être posées les conditions biologiques de la génération. Jamais il n'est permis de séparer ces divers aspects au point d'exclure positivement soit l'intention procréatrice, soit le rapport conjugal. La relation, qui unit le père et la mère à leur enfant, prend racine dans le fait organique et plus encore dans la démarche délibérée des époux, qui se livrent l'un à l'autre et dont la volonté de se donner s'épanouit et trouve son aboutissement véritable dans l'être qu'ils mettent au monde." Ibid., 470.

[41] "Sur ce point également, on Nous a demandé de donner quelques directives. Au sujet des tentatives de fécondation artificielle humaine "in vitro" qu'il Nous suffise d'observer qu'il faut les rejeter comme immorales et absolument illicites." Ibid., 471.

1.2.4. Allocution to Participants at the Seventh International Congress of Haematology, 12 September 1958

Once again, in another encounter with medical professionals in blood treatment, Pius XII makes recourse to his previous teaching regarding human artificial fertilization. He observes that human condition due to hereditary problem sometimes places married couples in procreative difficulty and so imposes the temptation to have a child by some morally illicit methods. In encouraging them on the teaching of the Church he notes that the Church is absolutely against these illicit methods of artificial insemination between people who are not married to each other, and equally between spouses.[42] Making reference to his previous teaching the Pope argues by saying that:

> …we condemn once again all types of artificial insemination, on the ground that this practice is not included among the rights of married couples and because it is contrary to the natural law and Catholic morals. As for artificial insemination between unmarried persons we declared in 1949 that this practice violates the principle of the natural law that new life may be procreated only in a valid marriage.[43]

From the foregoing, we can see that the Pope has been consistent in condemning artificial means of procreation which substitutes for the conjugal act but approving of the means whose role is to assist the conjugal act to realize its natural end. In addition, in this last discourse the Pope recommends adoption as a morally licit and legal method of having a child by married couples diagnosed to be infertile and who cannot have their condition medically treated in a morally licit way.

The summary of Pius XII's teaching contained in his discourses regarding human artificial fertilization as seen above could be outlined in five points:

---

42 Pius XII, *Allocution to Participants at the Seventh International Congress of Hematology*, 12 September 1958: in *AAS* 50 (1958): 732–748.

43 Ibid. "… pour réprouver à nouveau toute espèce d'insémination artificielle, parce que cette pratique n'est pas comprise dans les droits des époux et qu'elle est contraire à la loi naturelle et à la morale catholique. Quant à l'insémination artificielle entre célibataires, déjà en 1949 Nous avions déclaré qu'elle violait le principe de droit natu- rel, que toute vie nouvelle ne peut être procréée que dans un mariage valide." 733.

1. Human artificial insemination cannot be treated exclusively or principally from only the biological and medical perspective and disregarding the natural moral law. The unity of the body and spiritual dimensions of the person must be taken into consideration in any moral decision on artificial procreation.
2. The generation of human life is limited to marriage; for this reason artificial insemination outside of marriage is to be condemned purely and simply.
3. The use of donor in the generation of human life is immoral and to be irrevocably condemned. The nature's design that, parents become two in one flesh is the only morally acceptable context from which children are fruits of such a union, and cannot be substituted by any other means. That is, the conjugal act as the most personal act of the couple should not be replaced in procreation.
4. Masturbation or other practice of obtaining germ cells outside sexual intercourse for insemination is always immoral because it contradicts the nature of marriage and of procreation and of the dignity of the person.
5. New methods cannot be excluded *a priori* on the ground of being new. The use of artificial means aimed either to facilitate the performance of the natural act or to bring about the natural act performed in a normal way to achieve its purpose.

1.3. The Teaching of Paul VI: *Humanae Vitae*, 25 July 1968

The encyclical *Humanae Vitae*[44] was released in a period of sexual revolution and extreme humanism. This was a time that the philosophical thought that favors unbridled veneration of the human body and all that calls for gratification was considered to be the true good of man. The tendency to desire or emphasize the bodily union of spouses without its corresponding procreation was being advocated. According to Catholic moral tradition, since Pius XII, inherent in marriage, are two fundamental dimensions of unity and procreation that are naturally inseparable. Therefore, any positive

---

44 Paul VI, Encyclical *Humanae Vitae*, 25 July 1968: in *AAS* 60 (1968): 486–492. The English version: (Boston MA: Pauline Books, 25 July 1968). Hereafter this encyclical will be cited as: *Humanae Vitae*.

attempt to separate one dimension from the other frustrates the true significance of marriage and thereby undermines the dignity of the spouses and contravening the moral law of God the author of marriage. This understanding is behind the teaching of Paul VI in *Humanae Vitae*. The basic argument of this document relevant to our enquiry is its principle of inseparability: that the unitive and the procreative meanings of the conjugal act must be kept together. Hence, the Pope avers, "each and every marriage act must remain open to the transmission of life."[45] In the light of this principle, Paul VI explains that:

> This particular doctrine, expounded on numerous occasions by the Magisterium, is based on the inseparable connection, established by God, which man on his own initiative may not break, between the unitive significance and the procreative significance which are both inherent to the marriage pact.[46]

The argument against contraception as presented by Paul VI in *Humanae Vitae* applies equally in the condemnation of artificial fertilization for the same reason of severance of the intrinsic connection between the two aspects of the conjugal act. As contraception violates the principle of inseparability of the conjugal act by seeking bodily union without procreation, so artificial fertilization *in vitro* or artificial insemination violates the same principle by seeking procreation without bodily relation. In contraception, only the unitive dimension of marriage is pursued at the detriment of the procreative. Likewise in artificial fertilization, the procreative meaning of marriage is desired, but the unitive aspect is frustrated or undermined. Ralph McInerny agrees that "it is this same principle that forbids separating the unitive from the procreative meanings in contraceptive sex and separating of the procreative from the unitive in homologous artificial fertilization,"[47] the principle that is operative in *Donum Vitae*. In either case, the essential nature of the marital act is deliberately hampered. Hence, the document insists that the intrinsic unity of love union and procreation must be maintained in each

---

45 Ibid., n. 11.
46 Ibid., n. 12.
47 Ralph McInerny, "*Humanae Vitae* and the Principle of Totality," in Janet E. Smith (ed.), *Why Humanae Vitae was Right: A Reader* (San Francisco: Ignatius Press, 1993), 329.

and every marital sexual activity even when it is foreseen to be infertile.⁴⁸ By this, Paul VI sees present in the marital act both the symbolic and functional senses implied in the procreative act, such that even when the act does not lead to a child, the symbolic sense of procreation is always inherent. Therefore, in either one or both senses, it would still show that in every sexual act of the couple there is the procreative dimension that should not be deliberately inhibited. It is true that it is not every sexual act that leads naturally to pregnancy or conception on account of some natural factors independent of the couple's will, for example the natural cycle in women which is an essential aspect of their sexual and procreative life. Indeed, the essence of the conjugal act carried out humanly and properly is not diminished by the fact of it not resulting in pregnancy. The conclusion reached on the problem of seeking procreation outside the conjugal act by the Catholic Magisterium would leave moral theologians and ethicists in years later to interpret the teaching of the Church and engage in a debate to ascertain the moral and right means to aid human procreation especially for couples with infertility challenges.

1.4. Opinions of Some Theologians

From the 20th century when biomedical practice came into a considerable theological discourse, there existed initially two sharp theological opinions on the question of artificial intervention in human procreation especially with regard to artificial insemination. The first opinion interprets the prohibition of artificial intervention on human procreation solely from the

---

48 Cf. *Humanae Vitae*, n. 11. Using the words of the document, the conjugal act of the couple "does not, moreover, cease to be legitimate even when, for reasons independent of their will, it is foreseen to be infertile. For its natural adaptation to the expression and strengthening of the union of husband and wife is not thereby suppressed. The fact is, as experience shows, that new life is not the result of each and every act of sexual intercourse. God has wisely ordered laws of nature and the incidence of fertility in such a way that successive births are already naturally spaced through the inherent operation of these laws. The Church, nevertheless, in urging men to the observance of the precepts of the natural law, which it interprets by its constant doctrine, teaches that each and every marital act must of necessity retain its intrinsic relationship to the procreation of human life."

perspective of the nature of the means employed. That is, the wrongness of the intervention depends on the means used to achieve conception. For example, when masturbation is involved. The second opinion however, considers any form of interference in the procreative process to be morally wrong. In other words, for this latter opinion, artificial insemination or IVF are intrinsically wrong means to achieve procreation because they are not the natural means to generate human life.[49] Although the controversy on the acceptability or morality of artificial procreation had always been there even before the 20th century when the Magisterium responded significantly to the problem. In fact, science and technology made it possible to intervene in the human procreative process with the development recorded in biomedicine. The question sent to the Congregation of the Inquisition in 1897 is indicative that there was already a controversy at that period. But, the official and authoritative condemnation of artificial insemination by Pius XII brought a new dimension to the whole debate.[50] However, there were theologians who disagreed with Pius XII's conclusion on artificial insemination and by extension IVF procedures at least the one that involves husband and wife. The Pope's condemnation of reproductive interventions outside the sexual act actually met some differing opinions from theologians including Catholic theologians.[51]

According to McCormick, for instance, Pius XII's interventions on the question of artificial procreation had two areas that are controversial among theologians: the authoritative character of the Pope's declarations and the issue of inseparability of the conjugal act. On the former, McCormick representing some theologians, feels that the Pope was addressing the problem on the official level for the first time after Leo XIII (many think that the negative answer from the Holy Office on artificial insemination at this time was founded on masturbation to obtain semen and so the debate prior to Pius XII was largely in view of this). Hence, the new dimension

---

49 Cf. Wakefield, *Artful Childmaking*, 38.
50 The debate on the question of human artificial procreation is a complex one. After Pius XII's series of discourses, theologians made efforts to determine the extent to which technology can intervene in human procreation. It was no longer a blanket condemnation or acceptance of technology as was the case previously.
51 Cf. McCormick, *The Critical* Calling, 335.

brought by Pius XII required a new interpretation. Little wonder some feel that the Church was at its initial stages of reflection, and so "it would be a disservice to attribute anything like a definitive character to Pius's conclusions."[52] These theologians seem to reason that the Pope's position on the matter was open for interpretations, evaluations and never to be taken for a definitive answer. This reasoning would lead McCormick to assert: "The basis of the rejection [*of IVF absolutely as illicit*] could be [most likely] the mere unnaturalness, or it could be that the Pontiff saw this as experimental and dangerous tampering with embryonic life."[53] Therefore, further development and improvement on the IVF procedure might alter its negative judgment. As for the later, regarding the meaning of the inseparability of the unitive and procreative dimensions of the conjugal act upon which the Pope condemns artificial interventions, some interpret Pius XII's condemnation to include IVF in all its forms.[54]

---

52 Ibid. On this point, McCormick receives support from the views of Ladislaus Orsy who thinks that the position of Pius XII at the time would not imply an exclusion of artificial insemination or IVF performed using the gamete cells of the couple. Cf. Laudislaus Orsy, "Reflections on the Text of a Canon," in *America* 154 (1986): 396–399; Giovanni B. Guzzetti, "Magistero della chiesa e fecundazione in vitro," in *Scuola Cattolica* 133 (1985): 284–299; Ibid., "Debolezza degli argomenti contro l'embryo-transfer," in *Rivista di teologia morale* 17 (1985): 71–79. McCormick cites Marcellino Zalba and Jan Visser as among renowned Catholic theologians who challenged Pius XII's condemnation of artificial insemination by husband based on the fact that it would be wrong to do so absolutely or to interpret the Pope as such. However, "Zalba regards the Papal analysis as to 'physicist,' leaning heavily on the materiality of the act and not enough on its moral significance. Visser acknowledges that we have come a long way from the days when papal allocution would forever end a discussion. He believes that the argument of Pius XII retains its value as a general principle but doubts its absoluteness where insemination by husband is involved." Cf. Marcellino Zalba, "Aspetti morali e giuridici circa l'inseminazione artificiale," in *Palestra del clero* 58 (1979): 438 ff; Jan Visser, "Problemi etici dell' embryo-transfer," in *Ricerca scientifica ed educazione permanente* 7, 9 (1982–1983): 47 ff.
53 McCormick, *The Critical Calling*, 335. (The emphasis is added).
54 See for example, Catholic Bishops of Victoria (Australia), *Submission to the Committee to Examine in Vitro Fertilization*, unpublished document, 6 August 1982. Cited in McCormick, *The Critical Calling*, 336. The document states, "in pursuit of the admirable end of helping an infertile couple to conceive and

However, there are some theologians who think that Pius XII's judgment on artificial insemination by husband and invariably homologous IVF is not clear. For them, *Humanae Vitae* as well as *Familiaris Consortio*'s exclusion of procreation without the unitive act as a doctrine borrowed from Pius XII cannot be sustained from the theological point of view. To this end William Daniel writes,

> All we learn from this passage of [*Humanae Vitae*], however, is that if the conjugal act is performed it should have these qualities: it should not be falsified in either of its essential 'significations.' This does not necessarily imply that if there is to be procreation it should be by means of a unitive act.[55]

This argument appears to be interesting, but it also seems to understand partially the reason for the document's conclusion. First, the thesis upon which this argument rests indicates, that from the moral point of view,

---

have their baby, I.V.F. intervenes in their supreme expression of mutual love. It separates 'baby-making' from 'lovemaking.'" It is this separation of the essential elements of marital union that constitutes the basic problem of IVF apart from other ethical problems with it. This point raised by the Australian bishops supports the teaching that IVF is morally wrong because it disconnects the unitive and the procreative aspects of the marital act that are naturally and essentially connected. McCormick makes reference to this work in order to criticize it because it acknowledges that IVF helps infertile couples to conceive, yet it is not judged morally licit. For McCormick, the principle of inseparability of the unitive and the procreative meanings in the conjugal act does not require that the generation of human life should not occur outside the conjugal act but that if there is a conjugal act it should not be broken. While the bishops limit the generation of new human life to the conjugal act, McCormick thinks that IVF does not break the principle since there would be no conjugal act to separate the two meanings inherent in it. Carlo Caffarra equally supports Pius XII's position by appealing to the same principle of inseparability to reject IVF: "The moral problem is that procreation can no longer be said to be – and in fact is not – dependent upon the sexual act between two married people" because of the active role of this procedure involving technical control. Ordinary, procreation as willed by God is the exclusive responsibility of the couple and not with the active role of the third person. See Carlo Caffarra, *L'Osservatore Romano* (4 July 1984): 5. Cited in McCormick, *The Critical Calling*, 336.

55 William Daniel, "In Vitro Fertilization: Two Problem Areas," in *Australian Catholic Record* 63 (1986): 21–31 at 31. See also: Daniel, "The Morality of in Vitro Fertilization," in Terence Kennedy (ed.), *Moral Studies* (Melbourne: Spectrum Publications, 1984), 47–71.

a child must be generated from the conjugal act. Meaning that the child should not be generated if not from the conjugal act. Therefore, generating a child outside the conjugal act is morally wrong. It seems clear to think that this does not invalidate the application of the principle of inseparability used in *Humanae Vitae* and in *Familiaris Consortio*[56] to artificial procreation. However, this would need to be done with the thesis that procreation should result only from the conjugal act; this indeed is an affirmation of the truth of man's nature and of God's will for procreation. But, Daniel, McCormick and others seem to have a different understanding of the inseparability of the unitive-procreative dimensions of sexual expression because they emphasize rather marital relationship in the context of responsibility for procreation as the only determining factor for procreation. In other words, the exclusion of AI or IVF based on the principle just stated would be theologically problematic to defend, so they claim.

The Magisterium's condemnation of techniques of artificial procreation does not refer to those methods that are designed to assist the conjugal act. From the beginning, generally speaking, Catholic moral theologians had always been united on the rejection of donor insemination, chiefly because it is deemed to be contrary to divine plan for marriage. Similarly, our interest at this point is limited to the opinions expressed on moral grounds after the formal speech of Pius XII as a magisterial position. Inasmuch as the Pope condemns artificial insemination or similar methods in a forceful way, his indication that infertile couples may utilize certain methods as aid to procreation, has opened the door for the debate on the nature of assistance to or substitution for the conjugal act. The new preoccupation of theologians consists in determining the conditions that can qualify for an aid to the conjugal act.

In the work of Father Edwin Healy entitled *Medical Ethics*, he sustains that the use of a syringe by the physician to project the semen toward the uterus after intercourse has been normally performed may be in line with the standard set by Pius XII. In his words:

> It is permissible for a physician, however, after husband and wife have rightly performed the marital act, artificially to propel the semen deposited in the vagina

---

[56] John Paul II, Apostolic Exhortation *Familiaris Consortio*, 22 November 1981.

into the uterus and fallopian tubes, for the physician's act in this case would consist merely in aiding nature... This process is rightly called, not artificial, but assistance, insemination.[57]

In *Medico-Moral Problems*, an impressive study undertaken by Gerald Kelly, in which he concerns himself with making the distinction between assisted and artificial insemination between the cervical spoon and the cervical cap, he makes some assumptions that are relevant to the debate. Donald DeMarco makes reference to him when he states that "the function of the cervical spoon is to aid sperm in their migration through the cervical os."[58] He states further: "obviously, this procedure is not artificial insemination in the ordinary sense of the expression; it is merely a technique for aiding marital intercourse to be fertile by overcoming certain physiological obstacles. Some might call it 'assisted insemination.'"[59] While Kelly would accept this technique to be an instance of assisted insemination, he considers the cervical method to be an example of artificial insemination and therefore a substitute for intercourse.[60] According to him, unlike the former technique that makes use of a cervical spoon, the cervical cap technique is carried out by obtaining the semen either by masturbation or by retrieval of semen after intercourse and placed in a cuplike container (the cap), and then lifted over the cervix. Kelly draws the conclusion that, on moral ground the former assists intercourse to achieve its end, which means it meets the standard for moral acceptability, but the latter replaces it with an artificial technique.

---

57 Edwin Healy, *Medical Ethics* (Chicago: Loyola University Press, 1956), 154. Cited in Donald DeMarco, *Biotechnology and the Assault on Parenthood* (San Francisco: Ignatius Press, 1991), 208. Healy by making attempt to distinguish between "artificial" and "assistance" appears to indicate that artificiality is negative. But it seems that the Pope does not reject what is artificial but what is against the nature of the conjugal act or replaces the essential act of procreation and that is the marital sexual act.
58 DeMarco, *Biotechnology and the Assault on Parenthood*, 208. The works of Kelly which DeMarco depends on are: Gerald Kelly, *Medico-Moral Problems*, Vol. II (St. Louis: The Catholic Hospital Association, 1957), 239–240; Kelly, "Artificial Insemination" in Charles E. Curran and Richard A. McCormick (eds.), *Dialogue About Catholic Sexual Teaching: Readings in Moral Theology* 8 (New Jersey: Paulist Press, 1993), 245.
59 Ibid.
60 Kelly, *Artificial Insemination*, 240.

Kelly further argues that: "if ejaculation into the vagina is not taken as the minimum norm of determining a natural sex act, there seems to be no sound way of determining such an act."[61] Kelly's statement here is critical of and opposed to the use of masturbation to obtain semen for artificial insemination. In the light of this, DeMarco indicates, that the use of a device such as a spoon, syringe or dilator to enable the sperm to move more readily toward the egg was approved by some moralists and canonists, namely, DeSmet, Merkelbach, Payen, and Ubach. The condition attached to their opinion suggests that exteriorizing the deposited semen from the vagina would make the procedure unacceptable.[62] Kelly claims that the majority opinion of theologians even before Pius XII declared openly that artificial insemination or similar technique of human procreation was illicit. Arguing that husband and wife have no right of procreating except through coitus. They think that coitus is the means established by nature, and the only means of procreation in keeping with human dignity and with the traditional notion of marriage contract. And so "... this majority opinion was that no substitute for conjugal intercourse is permissible."[63] The contrary view, simply known as "a minority opinion," had it that "the right of a validly married couple to generate children is not limited to intercourse but might include the use of artificial means not in itself immoral."[64] This minority opinion emphasized the right of the married couple to procreate children by any medical means available to them insofar as the means is not unlawful in itself. This opinion considered insemination to be licit if the husband's semen is obtained outside the coitus but without the unnatural stimulation of the sexual faculty that has the quality of masturbation that was explicitly condemned by the Magisterium. The examples of such non-stimulating methods are the removal of semen from testicles or epididymis by aspiration or from seminal vesicles by massage.[65] By this it seems clear that the minority opinion in principle accepts procreation outside coitus

---

61 Ibid., 247.
62 Cf. Wakefield, *Artful ChildMaking*, 44; DeMarco, *Biotechnology and the Assault on Parenthood*, 209.
63 Kelly, *Artificial Insemination*, 248.
64 Ibid.
65 Kelly, *Medico-Moral Problems*, 18.

if the act of procuring the gamete for insemination is not immoral *per se*. It is difficult here following the magisterial teaching to identify the means other than the coital act that can be morally right. Simply understood, according to Kelly, while the majority opinion maintained that the conjugal act must be the source of conception, the minority opinion instead emphasized marriage relationship in totality to be the criterion for procreation. This distinction between the majority and minority opinions of theologians is indicated in the thoughts of Kelly but more pronounced in the work of Wakefield.[66]

John Mahoney in *Bioethics and Belief*[67] expresses the views of the so-called minority opinion, the theological position that still exists even after Pius XII's reprobation of artificial insemination and in vitro fertilization. Generally, discussions on human artificial fertilization in the 1970s and following years prior to the publication of *Donum Vitae* were centered on the issues of the morality of experimentation on the human embryo,

---

66 Cf. Ibid; Wakefield, *Artful Childmaking*.
67 This work first published in *Bioethics and Belief* in 1984 has also appeared in *Dialogue About Catholic Sexual Teaching: Readings in Moral Theology* n. 8, edited by Charles E. Curran and Richard A. McCormick (New York: Paulist Press, 1993), 251–266. In this work, Mahoney having made an impressive evaluation of the Church's teaching on artificial insemination and artificial fertilization *in vitro* concludes, that in principle there is nothing morally wrong about resorting to artificial insemination by the husband or to in vitro fertilization within a marriage if the husband and wife provide the genetic materials. He claims that the technology of artificial fertilization could be morally good and desirable because in itself it is morally neutral. "… if science can now bring to birth this loving expression of the love between husband and wife which would otherwise simply not exist, *because of the absence of children*, this too, it would appear, must be seen as part of the Creator's loving plan for all his children." Ibid., 257. (The emphasis is added); Marcellino Zalba, "Aspetti morali e giuridici circa l'inseminazione artificiale," in *Palestra del clero* 58 (1979): 438; Jan Visser, "Problemi etici dell'embryo-transfer," in *Ricerca scientifica ed educazione permanente* 7–9 (1982–1983): 47; Patrick Verspieren, "L'Aventure de la fécundation in vitro," in *Etudes* (1982): 479–492; Richard A. McCormick, *How Brave a New World: Dilemmas in Bioethics* (Garden City, New York: Doubleday, 1981), 308–312; Johannes Gründel, "Zeungung in der Retorte-unsittlich?" in *Stimmen der Zeit* 103 (1978): 675–682; Charles E. Curran, *Politics, Medicine, and Christian Ethics* (Philadelphia: Fortress, 1973), 200–219.

risks to the child to be born, negative consequences on the institution of marriage and family, exploitative effects on women and the changing image of parenthood and social values, these have since become the preoccupation in biomedical and theological debates. Hence, the publication of the Instruction *Donum Vitae* by the Congregation for the Doctrine of the Faith to make some evaluations on this all-important matter regarding human life and nature of the transmission of this life remains a significant development. And to this document we now turn.

B. An Overview of the Instruction *Donum Vitae*

1.1. The Instruction's Three Lines of Argument against Artificial Fertilization

The purpose of this section is basically to study the argumentation and significance of *Donum Vitae* in the evaluation of the simple case IVF.[68] The insights from the document will guide us to apply the principles of the Church's teaching particularly as it relates to the simple case in subsequent

---

[68] It can be recalled that at the end of the nineteenth century, the Church's Magisterium through the Holy See at the time known as the Holy Office (*Congregatio Sancti Ufficii*) now changed to the Congregation for the Doctrine of the Faith, made the first unsubstantiated negative response *(Non Licere*, 17 March 1897) to the question on artificial insemination. This position was confirmed and substantiated by Pius XII in his discourse of 29 September 1949 to the Fourth International Congress of Catholic Physicians, in *AAS* 41 (1949): 557–561 and by John XXIII on 15 May 1961, in the encyclical *Mater et Magistra* (*AAS* 53 [1961]: 447). It is equally worthy of note that the argument of *Humanae Vitae*, n. 12 against artificial contraception and which underscores the fact, that the morality of human procreation requires the biological integrity of the sexual act, was employed fully by *Donum Vitae*. And because *Donum Vitae* is in accord and continuity with the recent magisterial doctrine on the dignity of human procreation and for the fact that it also establishes the foundational and deeper argument against the simple case, it justifies our attention on its use for our study on this problem. The preceding comment is relevant in respect to the newer Instruction *Dignitas Personae* of 2008, which is essentially an update to the former and does not really raise any new judgment/dimension on the simple case. For this reason, we will not pay much attention to it but sparingly make reference to it where necessary.

sections of the work.[69] The Instruction *Donum Vitae* renews the Church's teaching on respect for human life, the sanctity of the conjugal union and the limits of biomedical and technological interventions in human procreation. It sets the criteria of moral judgment as regards the applications of scientific research and technology, especially as it concerns human life in its beginnings. The foundations of the arguments of the document are derived from the Sacred Scripture, natural law, Church's moral tradition and scientific facts. The Instruction marks a significant development in the magisterial teaching on artificial procreation. It is divided into three principal parts with an introduction and a conclusion. In the light of John Paul II's thoughts, theologians like William E. May have indicated that *Donum Vitae*'s message is weaved with three principal lines of argument on artificial procreation, namely, argument from the principle of inseparability of the conjugal act, the "language of the body" and the "begotten not made."[70] Let us briefly examine these points of reasoning below.

1.1.1. The Principle of Inseparability of the Conjugal Act

The argument on the unbreakable link between conjugal union and procreation that the document advances, makes clear the true meaning of marriage as an enduring unitive and procreative relationship. On the section treating homologous artificial fertilization, *Donum Vitae* recalls the Church's teaching from the moral point of view on the connection between bodily relation and procreation as intrinsic dimensions of the conjugal act. The Instruction affirms the teaching of Paul VI when it argues that there is a personal and natural connection in the process of procreation which must remain tied together to make the generation of human life truly worthy of man and in accordance to God's plan. In other words, the Magisterium once again affirms the truth that there is:

> Inseparable connection, willed by God and unable to be broken by man on his own initiative, between the two meanings of the conjugal act: the unitive meaning and the procreative meaning. Indeed, by its intimate structure, the conjugal act

---

69 The review of the document, *Donum Vitae* which we undertake here will be limited to the aspects that could be applied to our central theme which is the simple case of in vitro fertilization and embryo transfer (IVF-ET).

70 Cf. May, *Catholic Bioethics and the Gift of Human Life*, 38–39.

> while most closely uniting husband and wife, capacitates them for the generation of new lives, according to laws inscribed in the very being of man and of woman.[71]

This moral teaching on inseparability as indicated above is dependent on the nature of the person as a composite being of body and spirit, inseparably united. The indication that the inseparable connection of the two meanings of the conjugal act is "unable to be broken by man on his own initiative," does not mean that it cannot be broken but that it should not be broken, it may not be separated, one aspect should not be sought with the intention of excluding the other, because they are meant to be together.

In fact, there are two actions working in tandem in the generation of human life: the personal act (moral act) and the act of nature (law of nature). The personal act of the couple in the act of procreation is the conjugal act and the act of nature is the natural process of conception obeying the law of nature. The Instruction acknowledges this truth when it states that:

> Indeed, by its intimate structure, the conjugal act, while most closely uniting husband and wife, capacitates them for the generation of new lives, according to laws inscribed in the very being of man and of woman.[72]

The fact of the unity of spouses and procreation as basic goods which result only from marriage is according to the natural law and the unity needed for the generation of new human life must be safeguarded. Expounding on the principle just quoted, *Donum Vitae* again appeals to the submission of *Humanae Vitae*:

> By safeguarding both these essential aspects, the unitive and the procreative, the conjugal act preserves in its fullness the sense of true mutual love and its ordination towards man's exalted vocation to parenthood.[73]

This doctrine of the Church precisely reveals the reason for the negative judgment of the Instruction regarding homologous in vitro fertilization and even in the so-called simple case IVF-ET. The separation of the goods of

---

71 *Humanae Vitae*, n. 12.
72 *Donum Vitae*, II, B/4. The principle recalls here was employed in the teaching of Paul VI in *Humanae Vitae*, n. 12.
73 Ibid.

love union and procreation creates an immoral context whereby either of the two meanings of the conjugal act is deliberately destroyed or forfeited. In so doing, it can have negative consequences on the couple and the new human life. Warning against homologous artificial fertilization, *Donum Vitae* stresses that:

> Homologous artificial fertilization, in keeping a procreation that is not the specific fruit of conjugal union, objectively effects an analogous separation between the goods and meanings of marriage.... Thus, fertilization is licitly sought when it is the result of a 'conjugal act that is ordered by its nature and by which the spouses become one flesh.' But from the moral point of view, procreation is deprived of its proper perfection when it is not desired as the fruit of the conjugal act, that is to say, of the specific act of the spouses' union.[74]

The teaching of the Instruction about the integrity of the conjugal act could be understood no less in the reasoning of Pius XII when he indicates that the marital act is not "a mere organic function for the transmission of the germs of life."[75] But that, it is "a personal action, a simultaneous natural self-giving which, in the words of Holy Scripture, effects the union in 'one flesh'... [and] implies a personal cooperation [of the spouses with God in giving new human life]."[76] In fact, the Instruction indicates that the conjugal act is a moral act, a personal act that unites and communicates spousal love on one hand and is at the same time open to the reception of

---

74 Ibid. The internal citation is from the *Code of Canon Law*, Can. 1061. This Canon states, "the conjugal act is that by which the marriage is consummated if the couple have performed (it) between themselves in a human manner." This statement making reference to the manner of performing the conjugal act, seems to suggest what W. E. May would think of when he makes the distinction between the genital act and the conjugal act. According W. E. May, the conjugal act is not simply a genital act between a man and a woman who happen to be married. It is in truth an act that inwardly participates in their marital union; it is an act inwardly participating in the "goods" of marriage, i.e., the good of steadfast fidelity and of exclusive marital love and the good of children. This being the case, the genital act is an imposed act by one of the spouses upon the other against reasonable desires of the other that violates the requirements of the moral order. Cf. William E. May, *Marriage: The Rock on Which the Family is Built*, 2nd Edition (San Francisco: Ignatius Press, 2009), 83–84.
75 Pius XII, *Address to the Italian Catholic Union of Midwives*. Cited in May, *Marriage*, 84.
76 Ibid.

new human life. The above teaching follows that procreation should not take place outside the conjugal act as it is done in IVF nor should sexual intercourse intentionally exclude the possibility of the gift of new life as in contraception.

In discussing the morality of artificial conception, the issue of contraception would seem inevitable to be touched. The reason is based on the link between contraception and artificial conception as the two moral issues that affect the conjugal act. In the same way as artificial fertilization offends the intrinsic connection of the marital act by circumventing it to achieve the generation of the child, so in its own way, contraception inhibits the generation of new life by blocking the unitive act from realizing its natural end. The Church has always taught that owing to the anthropological structure of the human person reflected in the nature of the conjugal act, "each and every act of conjugal intercourse must remain open to the possibility of new life."[77] The deliberate intention to frustrate the realization of the gift of new life by a human act is considered in the mind of the Church as an illicit act. In an intelligent work published by Cormac Burke, one can find a convincing reason to see why contraception is illicit. According to him, contraceptive sexual relation between spouses can be self-assertive, it expresses the selfishness of the spouses because each one is seeking himself or herself and failing truly to find or know or give the other. This attitude is contrary to the principle of marital love which naturally tends towards perpetuation of the couple in conjugal bond. In fact, "... it is the case of two persons in love, who naturally want to perpetuate the love that draws them to one another, so that they can have the joy of seeing it take flesh in a new life, fruit of that mutual spiritual and carnal knowledge by which they express their spousal love."[78] There seems to be no better way to perpetuate the memory of self-giving in marriage than to allow consciously that most significant love act the possibility of generating a new life.

---

77 *Humanae Vitae*, n. 14.
78 Cormac Burke, "Children and Values," in Russell E. Smith (ed.), *Trust the Truth: A Symposium on the Twentieth Anniversary of the Encyclical Humanae Vitae* (Braintree: Massachusetts, The Pope John XXIII Medical-Moral Research and Education Center, 1988), 361.

Paul VI defines contraception as "any action which either before, at the moment of, or after marital intercourse, is specifically intended to impede procreation – whether as an end or a means."[79] In these words the Pope considers the act of contraception not purely as an external act but equally the positive intention to hinder the possibility of new life of a child which might result from that marital intercourse. Pope John Paul II describes this teaching as "a teaching which belongs to the permanent patrimony of the Church's moral doctrine. The uninterrupted continuity with which the Church has taught it derives from her responsibility for the true good of the human person, of the human person of the spouses, first of all, for conjugal love is their most precious good."[80] *Donum Vitae* acknowledges the link between contraception and artificial conception in its treatment of the principle of the conjugal act. It sees an intrinsic connection between the goods of spousal lovemaking and life generation; the principle of the conjugal act requires that this connection remains intact in the exercise of marital rights. As the document indicates, contraception frustrates the conjugal act of its openness to procreation and by so doing causes a deliberate disconnection of the ends of marriage.[81] Contraception acts against the specific laws, the capacity God the Creator has established in human nature to be exercised in marriage. Hence, contraception like artificial conception constitutes a moral problem in marriage. Contraception carries the same moral problem of being intrinsically evil as *in vitro* fertilization.

1.1.2. The "Language of the Body" Argument

Human body communicates symbolically and this is more evident in matters of sexuality. There is an inherent attraction between the masculine and feminine genders seeking a sort of completion of their being through communion. This experience has foundation in the nature of the human person. Indeed, the anthropological-theological structure of the human person created by God in his peculiarity of body and spiritual soul composition reveals

---

79 *Humanae Vitae*, n. 14.
80 John Paul II, *Discourse to Participants at the Fourth International Congress for the Family of Europe and of Africa* (Vatican City: Libreria Editrice Vaticana, 14 March 1988). This can be found in www.vatican.va
81 Cf. *Donum Vitae*, II/B, 4, a.

his dignity that cannot be attributed to other animals. This is contrary to some held views that the soul and the body are two separable entities in the manner that the soul is imprisoned in the body.[82] This latter school of thought considers the body of the person as a biological or physical entity that could be subjected to physical laws alone. Marriage as a committed relationship between a man and a woman, two persons of bodies and souls becoming two in one body, this reality has some implications and moral significance. It is not the unity of simple material bodies, but a relationship that transcends the physical and social order.

The theological and moral meaning of marital relationship is explained in consideration of the "language of the body" symbolism. Marriage expresses the bodily and spiritual self-giving of the spouses, mutually to each other in an enduring relationship that is at once unitive and procreative. Following *Donum Vitae*,

> The moral value of the intimate link between the goods of marriage and between the meanings of the conjugal act is based upon the unity of the human being, a unity involving bodily and spiritual soul. Spouses mutually express their personal love in the 'language of the body,' which clearly involves both 'spousal meanings' and parental ones.[83]

---

82 Platonic dualism tries to force man to believe that the soul was "in" the body in roughly the same manner that a pilot is in his ship. The originator of this theory, Plato would never know the implication of his theory as manifested in Technology attempting to dominate the human person without considering his intrinsic worth as a created being with a difference, a compound being of bodily and spiritual dimensions. Aristotle, after Plato was right in his attempt to correct this theory by affirming the essential unity of body and soul of the human person. Many centuries later, St. Thomas Aquinas, defending the Aristotelian theory, expounded the body-spirit relationship in terms of the unity of both. (See his *Summa Contra Gentiles*, II. C. 68). It is with the Aquinas' analysis that the Church defined the soul as the substantial form of the human body (Council of Vienne, 1312; DS 902). The point to note therefore is that the body is not to be treated as an object, a thing that can be manipulated as it is suspected or viewed in artificial fertilization *in vitro*.

83 *Donum Vitae*, B/4, b. The description of the human person as being body and soul affirms the teaching of the Fathers of the Second Vatican Council on the Church in the Modern World. Cf. Pastoral Constitution *Gaudium et Spes*, n. 14. The internal citation is taken from John Paul II, *General Audience* (16 January 1980), in *Insegnamenti di Giovanni Paolo II*, III, I (1980): 148–152.

As *Donum Vitae* makes us to understand, the constitution of the human person is such that he is both spiritual and bodily. He is not simply a material body and not purely a spiritual being, but a compound of body and soul inseparably. The Instruction affirms the significance of the body when it says that:

> It is in their bodies and through their bodies that the spouses consummate their marriage and are able to become father and mother. In order to respect the language of their bodies and their mutual generosity, the conjugal union must take place with respect for its openness to procreation; and the procreation of the person must be the fruit of the result of married love.[84]

The importance of the above quotation is found with the insistence that "fertilization achieved outside the bodies of the couple remain by this very fact deprived of the meanings and the values which are expressed in the language of the body and in the union of human persons."[85] Indeed, one may say, to intentionally exclude either marital sexual union or procreation from marriage is to falsify the "language of the body" spoken in marital relationship. Its wrongness lies in a kind of deception because the body naturally speaks the truth. So, just as excluding the procreative dimension of the conjugal act through contraceptive choices is wrong, so also excluding the unitive dimension from the choice to procreate is wrong. As some theologians indicate, "Conjugal communion is not simply a union of bodies, much less of gametes. On the contrary, it is an interpersonal union, one that involves body and spirit…. Conjugal communion is inseparably spiritual as well as corporeal."[86] Therefore, procreation would be proper to the dignity of the person when it is achieved as a result of the unity of the bodily and spiritual self-giving of the spouses in conjugal sexual intercourse and not otherwise. According to this argument, the simple case IVF-ET, insofar as conception is sought outside the sexual act of the spouses,

---

84 *Donum Vitae*, II, B/4, b. For further reading: John Paul II, *Discourse to those taking part in the 35th General Assembly of the World Medical Association*, 29 October 1983: *AAS* 76 (1984): 393.
85 Ibid.
86 David Q. Liptak and Leo T. Duffy, *The Gift of Life: A Theological Commentary on the Vatican 'Instruction on Respect for Human Life in its origin and on the Dignity of Procreation'* (Lake Worth: Liturgical Publications, 1988), 54.

remains immorally wrong and unacceptable. The good intention of the spouses to have a child and the efficiency of the technique cannot justify the replacement of the sexual act as the only suitable font of the child's life.

1.1.3. The "Begotten-Not-Made" Argument

In Catholic moral doctrine, the respect for human life does not begin only after the birth of the child but from the moment of conception through the different stages of development. It means that the origin of human life is equally significant as when that life is brought into existence at birth. The prenatal human being deserves the respect due to every human person by virtue of its ontological nature as a human being. In the light of this doctrine, *Donum Vitae* declares that:

> In his unique and irrepeatable origin, the child must be respected and recognised as equal in personal dignity to those who give him life. The human person must be accepted in his parents' act of union and love; the generation of the child must therefore be the fruit of that mutual giving which is realized in the conjugal act wherein the spouses cooperate as servants and not as masters in the work of the Creator who is love.[87]

The role of spouses in procreation therefore should flow from the desire to be God's obedient servants who simply respond to God's invitation to be agents through which new human life is brought forth into the world. This responsibility as parents excludes the usurpation of the Creator's absolute authority over life. This suggests why the document uses the right verb "cooperate" to describe the role of the parents in human procreation. Parents, according to this understanding cannot decide on their own to violate the natural means provided by the Creator for the generation of human life. They must respect the conjugal act and act according to the moral law inscribed in them by virtue of being rational beings.

Furthermore, it is to be underscored as the document clearly states:

> ... the origin of a human person is the result of an act of giving. The one conceived must be the fruit of his parents' love. He cannot be desired or conceived as the product of an intervention of medical or biological techniques; that would be equivalent to reducing him to an object of scientific technology.[88]

---

87 Ibid., II/4, c.
88 Ibid. The internal citation makes reference to *Gaudium et Spes,* n. 51.

As quoted, the means of bringing into existence human life must be in accord with the inestimable value or dignity of the human person. The desire for a child is in itself noble and praiseworthy. Yet, the means to achieve this desire should not undermine or give a wrong impression about the child to be begotten. Inasmuch as biomedical science and scientific technology constitute valuable assets to ease man's struggles and wellbeing, they should not be used against human life or his dignity. Artificial fertilization *in vitro* or artificial insemination which involves some exercise of professional decision on which embryo to live or be discarded, introduces a situation of absolute control over human life, an authority which belongs only to God. This implies that intervention in human procreation should exclude the choice and means of absolute control and dominion.[89] The manipulative nature of technology and the professional function of technicians in the so-called simple case IVF-ET remain suspicious for other reasons apart from substituting for the sexual act.

Furthermore, *Donum Vitae* emphasizes that:

> The moral relevance of the link between the meanings of the conjugal act and between the goods of marriage, as well as the unity of the human being and the dignity of his origin, demand that the procreation of the human person be brought about as the fruit of the conjugal act specific to the love between spouses.[90]

It is important to consider the fact that human beings are creatures with inestimable worth, and so the means by which they come into the world cannot have the same significance with those of other animals. There is an anthropological and moral relevance to insist that human procreation naturally has and should have its source in the conjugal act. The life of the new child who comes into the world deserves respect even before his birth. This follows the teaching of the document that human beings are *subjects* and not *objects*, and so, they are to be *begotten*, not made. They are persons not products.

In summarizing the three lines of argument employed in *Donum Vitae*, and as exposed above, it would be profitable to make recourse to Ratzinger. He expresses the truth of man's inviolable worth better, when as the

---

89 Ibid.
90 Ibid.

President of the Congregation for the Doctrine of the Faith, needing to unveil the Instruction explains, that the correct vision of man entails three theses: (1) the human body is a constitutive part of the human person and expresses itself through it; (2) the human person is endowed with such dignity that he or she can never be dismissed merely as a "thing," an "object"; on the contrary, the human person must always be acknowledged as a "subject" – "someone" and not "something"; (3) the only act which, of its very nature, is ethically worthy of a new human life, is the conjugal act.[91] These tripartite anthropological and moral views suggest that the generation of new human life should be in accord with the intrinsic dignity of human life and must respect the order of nature ordained by God the Creator. It is within these criteria that the simple case of homologous IVF-ET receives its negative judgment in *Donum Vitae*.

1.2. Moral Principles of *Donum Vitae*

The document identifies the life of the human being and the special nature of the transmission of human life as the two fundamental values connected with the techniques of human procreation. The moral evaluation of any technique of artificial procreation must be based on the respect, safety and preservation of these values. In the light of these basic principles mentioned, we shall treat in this section some relevant considerations where these principles reflect in the Instruction.

1.2.1. *The Life of the Human Being*

Human life begins at conception. Human life called into being in the world has different stages of development that commence when the ovum of a woman is properly fertilized by the sperm of the man. This significant event initiates the beginning of human life and once begun deserves the respect and protection due to every human person without prejudice. Sgreccia

---

91 Cf. Charles Connolly (ed.), *New Life: Church Teaching on Technology and Fertilization, with Commentaries* (Dublin: Four Courts Press, 1987), 12; *L'Osservatore Romano*, English edition, 16 March 1987), 8. Cited in Liptak and Duffy, *The Gift of Life,* 2.

succinctly describes the phenomenon of human life by comparing it with other created living beings in the world. For him, life in the world

> ... in its unfolding in various forms throughout the world, has its summit in the life of man: even for biologists and naturalists, man constitutes the richest, most independent, and most active form of life, at the highest level of the kingdom of living things and the peak of the natural history of the universe.... As for medicine, its central goal is service to man and his health.[92]

This postulation corresponds to the vision of *Donum Vitae* about human life:

> Physical life, with which the course of human life in the world begins, certainly does not itself contain the whole of a person's value, nor does it represent the supreme good of man who is called to eternal life. However it does constitute in a certain way the 'fundamental' value of life, precisely because upon this physical life all the other values of the person are based and developed.[93]

The Instruction recognizes that the inviolable innocent human life "from the moment of conception until death is a sign and requirement of the very inviolability of the human person to whom the Creator has given the gift of life."[94] The value of human life constitutes therefore one of the reference points upon which those engaged in the simple case laboratory fertilization must evaluate their action. Would the human life in its most vulnerable state be accorded the deserved reverence and protection in this technology of human procreation? Does the inherent dignity of human life not being impaired or undermined in the use of the simple case IVF-ET technology? These are some of the questions that must apply in the decision to have a child by means of the simple case and other forms of medical assisted technology. The Church is aware of the risks usually associated with IVF technology and would insist that those who make the choice for this form of technology realize that the human life they deal with is not something as *object* but someone, a *subject* creature of God the Creator, with inherent values that transcend the physical world.

It is informative that the document highlights for reflection the life of the human being owing to the fact that most frequently, and indeed

---

92 Sgreccia, *Personalistic Bioethics*, 105.
93 *Donum Vitae*, Introd., 4.
94 Ibid. The citation makes reference to John Paul II, *Discourse to those taking part in the 35th General Assembly of the World Medical Association*, 1983.

unfortunately, in the use of technology for procreation, medicine seems to "treat the body as a mere complex of tissues and organs."[95] Medicine is often accused of treating the human body and worse still, the human embryo as means to an end. It fails to recognize that the body of the human being is both a spiritual and bodily reality, a being of a unified totality. That is why the Instruction teaches that the nature of the human being should be considered when one decides to engage in artificial fertilization because he would not be dealing with only cells but the entire person, both of the child to be born and the woman as the mother. Otherwise, technology would not simply be assisting the infertile couple to have a child but exercising dominion over the process of procreation and the life of the child and that of his mother.

1.2.2. Marriage as the Only Licit Context for Procreation

By virtue of the unique nature of human life, which we briefly described above, the Instruction observes that the only context suitable for the generation and nurturing of human life is marriage. The means of the transmission of human life is a value with a profound moral and theological relevance. The truth of this assertion is seen in the thoughts of John XXIII. *Donum Vitae* affirms his teaching on this matter when it states that:

> The transmission of human life is entrusted by nature to a personal and conscious act as such is subject to the all-holy laws of God: immutable and inviolable laws which must be recognized and observed. For this reason one cannot use means and follow methods which could be licit in the transmission of the life of plants and animals.[96]

---

95 Paul Lauritzen, "Whose Bodies? Which Selves? Appeals to Embodiment in Assessments of Reproductive Technology," in M. Therese Lysaught and Joseph J. Kotva Jr. (eds.), *On Moral Medicine: Theological Perspectives in Medical Ethics*, 3rd Edition (Michigan/Cambridge: Grand Rapids, 2012), 851.

96 *Donum Vitae, Introd.*, 4; John XXIII, *Encyclical Mater et Magistra*, 15 May 1961: in *AAS* 53 (1961): 447. The original text: "Quoniamque hominis vita aliis hominibus consulto et cogitate traditur, sequitur idcirco, ut hoc agatur ad Dei praescriptiones sanctissimas, firmissimas, inviolatas; quas scilicet nemo non agnoscere, non servare debet. Quocirca in hac re nemini omnium licet omnium licet iis uti viis rationibusque, quibus vel arborum vel animantium vita propagare licet."

This holds true and recalls the fact that the use of technology for human artificial fertilization was initially developed for animal husbandry.[97] The concern in artificial procreation cannot be centered only on the issue of nurturing the new life already brought into the world, it is equally very significant to evaluate the means by which the new human life is conceived and born. In this sense, it is not simply a matter of biological or social consideration but equally a matter with anthropological and theological relevance. *Donum Vitae* teaches that the acts of begetting and nurturing are properly and naturally situated in marital union. With this, parenthood assumes a responsibility in the creative-nurturing act of God. The Magisterium acknowledges the "power" of advanced technology to reproduce human beings asexually outside the context of marital union, but it warns: "what is technically possible is not for that very reason morally admissible."[98] Therefore, the Instruction declares the need to engage in a deep reflection on the fundamental values of life and of human procreation as an indispensable tool in formulating a moral evaluation of such technological interventions on a human procreation from the first stages of the development of the human being.

The Vatican document asks the pertinent question of why human procreation must take place in marriage. In its response, it states that:

> Every human being is always to be accepted as a gift and blessing of God. However, from the moral point of view a truly responsible procreation vis-à-vis the unborn child must be the fruit of marriage.[99]

In this quotation, the document seems to recognize the fact that there are some children who are born outside the marital union or by means other than through the conjugal act. Notwithstanding the wrong means through which they were born, they are to be received as God's gift and a blessing of God. It therefore reminds us of the morally licit context of begetting the child and that is marriage. The teaching of the Second Vatican document is recalled to substantiate this view thus: "... the procreation of a new person, whereby the man and the woman collaborate with the power of

---

97 Sgreccia, *Personalist Bioethics*, 495.
98 *Donum Vitae*, Introd., 4.
99 Ibid., II, A/1.

the Creator, must be the fruit and the sign of the mutual self-giving of the spouses, of their love and of their fidelity."[100] The Instruction goes further to point out that the child born in marriage is to the parents a confirmation and completion of their mutual self-giving. The child is the living image of their love, the permanent sign of their conjugal union, the living and indissoluble expression of their paternity and maternity.[101] This goes to confirm why the use of technology to replace that most intimate and personal act of conjugal love that the child symbolizes for the parents is morally wrong.

1.2.3. The Dignity of Human Procreation

The transmission of human life has its special character because from the beginning it involves a creative act of God. By virtue of this, man stands in a special relationship with God his Creator. Again, the dignity of human procreation is related to the inviolable worth of human life and the integrity of the conjugal act. The communion of love and life of the spouses is fundamental to underscore the dignity of human procreation. This communion reflects the relationship that exists in the Divine Trinity and equally a symbol of God's relationship with man. As the Instruction rightly points out:

> God, who is love and life, has inscribed in man and woman the vocation to share in a special way in his mystery of personal communion and in his work as Creator and Father. For this reason marriage possesses specific goods and values in its union and in procreation which cannot be likened to those existing in lower forms of life. Such values and meanings are of the personal order and determine from the moral point of view the meaning and limits of artificial interventions on procreation and on the origin of human life.[102]

In fact, given that man shares in the image and likeness of God, and for that very reason is able to share in the vocation to transmit new human life, this reveals where human procreation derives its dignity. Biblically, the attention and act with which God created man would remain meaningful theologically and anthropologically in the discussion of human procreation.

---

100 Ibid. Reference is made to *Gaudium et Spes*, n. 50.
101 Ibid. The internal citation is from: John Paul II, Apostolic Exhortation *Familiaris Consortio*, n. 14.
102 Ibid., 3.

John Paul II would want us to return to the biblical accounts for a proper appreciation of the significance of marriage and its role in procreation. This is what he intended to achieve in his famous catechesis developed into his *Theology of the Body*.[103] Properly speaking, marriage is a human act, a human act because the man and woman who agree to marry do so in freedom and full knowledge. Being a human act does not suggest its origin but its object. God is the origin of marriage. The Priestly tradition of the creation narrative shows that: "God created man [*ha'adam*] in his image; in the divine image he created him; male and female he created them. God blessed them: saying: 'Be fertile and multiply; fill the earth and subdue it. Have dominion over the fish of the sea, the birds of the air, and all the living things that move on the earth'" (Gen. 1, 27–28).[104]

We make efforts to elaborate on the dignity of human procreation in order to show that human procreation has a special character because it is about the life of an inviolable human being in close relationship with God besides its unique and amazing constitution. It is about a human being of a particular identity, with inalienable rights and more so, human life is the fruit of mutual love of persons who have made themselves worthy to receive the gift of life. Indeed, the integrity and sanctity of conjugal union require that procreation must correspond to other values of life and marital union.

1.2.4. Biomedical Technology as a Gift in the Service of Life

The first section of the Instruction centers on biomedical research and the teaching of the Church on the anthropological and moral identity of the human person. This document invites man to appreciate the inestimable value of human life that is a gift of God (Ps. 127, 3) in reference to the challenges posed by recent biomedical research. The Magisterium in this document reiterates the responsibility with which man must assume with respect to interventions on human procreation considering the ambivalent nature of contemporary biomedical technologies. The benefits which science and technology offer man are numerous but when it is used

---

103 John Paul II, *Man and Woman He Created Them: A Theology of the Body*, Trans. Michael Waldstein (Boston MA: Pauline Books and Media, 2006), 136.
104 Ibid.,

improperly without adequate evaluation, it could turn to destroy man who manufactures it. And so, it is indicated that the magisterial intervention in this issue is not on the grounds of any particular competence in the discipline of experimental sciences, rather, by virtue of her vocation. The document declares the intention of the Church when it says that:

> It intends to put forward, by virtue of its evangelical mission and apostolic duty, the moral teaching corresponding to the dignity of the person and to his or her integral vocation. It intends to do so by expounding the criteria of moral judgment as regards the applications of scientific research and technology, especially in relation to human life and its beginnings.[105]

In fact, the Church's Magisterium is never in doubt of the positive contributions of science and technology and what it can do to improve the quality of human life. Hence, the document acknowledges with gratitude the contributions science and technology make to benefit the human person when it observes:

> Science and technology are valuable resources for man when placed at his service and when they promote his integral development for the benefit of all; but they cannot of themselves show the meaning of existence and of human progress. Being ordered to man, who initiates and develops them, they draw from the person and his moral values the indication of their purpose and the awareness of their limits.[106]

Thus, according to *Donum Vitae* science and technology cannot claim to be morally neutral. Indeed, the criteria for guidance in scientific research cannot come from mere technical efficiency, not from research's possible usefulness to some human beings at the expense of others, nor does it come from prevailing ideologies. Instead, they need to come from some basic moral criteria which respect the inalienable rights of the human person according to God's design, in order that their service to man may be truly valuable and good for him.[107] The Instruction notes that the rapid development of technological discoveries gives greater urgency to this need to respect the criteria of the moral law, because science without conscience can only lead to man's ruin. Consequently, it recalls that: "Our era needs

---

105 *Donum Vitae*, Introd.,1.
106 Ibid., 2.
107 Ibid.

such wisdom more than bygone ages if discoveries made by man are to be further humanized. For the future of the world stands in peril unless wiser people are forthcoming."[108] The wisdom needed as suggested by the Instruction is to follow the principle that what is technically possible is not for that very reason morally admissible. Rather, the technology that serves man in his integrality, that assists the conjugal act and respect human life may be morally encouraged.

1.2.5. Donum Vitae *on the Simple Case IVF-ET*

In the section of the Instruction dealing with homologous artificial fertilization, the document asks: "Is homologous 'in vitro' fertilization morally licit?" The prompt answer to this question is located within the three lines of argument presented in the preceding section. These arguments are based on the affirmation of: (1) the inseparable connection between the unitive and procreative meanings of the conjugal act; (2) the unity (the desire for communion, mutual self donation and reception of each other) of the couple as human persons in their bodily and spiritual dimensions (commonly called the "language of the body") involving both "spousal meanings" and "parental ones" well taught by John Paul II; and (3) the dignity of the person in his personal identity and his unique origin.

With the above stated perspectives, the Instruction reasons that homologous artificial fertilization cannot be morally accepted. According to the document, nature requires that "the procreation of a human person be brought about as the fruit of the conjugal act specific to the love between spouses."[109] The link between procreation and the conjugal act is thus shown to be of great importance on the anthropological and moral planes, and it throws light on the positions of the Magisterium with regard to homologous artificial fertilization.[110] To apply the above teaching to the question of the simple case that we are discussing, *Donum Vitae* gives an affirmation to the position of Pius XII on the relevance of safeguarding the unitive and procreative meanings of the conjugal act. To be precise, it states:

---

108 Ibid., Introd., 3. The internal citation is from *Gaudium et Spes*, n. 15; Paul VI, *Populorum Progressio*, n. 20: in *AAS* 59 (26 March 1967): 267.
109 Ibid.
110 Ibid.

It is never permitted to separate these different aspects to such a degree as positively to exclude either the procreative intention (like in *contraception*) or the conjugal relation (*artificial procreation in vitro*).[111]

Donum Vitae therefore concludes that:

> Fertilization is licitly sought when it is the result of a 'conjugal act which is per se suitable for the generation of children to which marriage is ordered by its nature and by which spouses become one flesh'. But from the moral point of view procreation is deprived of its proper perfection when it is not desired as the fruit of the conjugal act, that is to say of the specific act of the spouses' union.[112]

Following this line of argument, the decision to have a child through the simple case IVF-ET, which occurs outside the conjugal act, is morally wrong and unacceptable. This is because, as the Church teaches, the intrinsic bond between the essential meanings (love union and procreation) of the conjugal act is separated in every form of IVF.

Secondly, the Instruction in considering the immorality of homologous artificial fertilization indicates that the dignity of the child is degraded. The reason being that the child is only to be begotten as the fruit of his parents love and not to be conceived as the

> Product of an intervention of medical or biological techniques; for that would be equivalent of reducing him to an object of scientific technology. No one may subject the coming of a child into the world to conditions of technical efficiency which are to be evaluated according to the standards of control and dominion.[113]

In fact, *Donum Vitae* insists,

> Conception in vitro is the result of the technical action which presides over fertilization. Such fertilization is neither in fact achieved nor positively willed as the expression and fruit of a specific act of the conjugal union. In homologous IVF and ET, therefore, even if it is considered in the context of '*de facto*' existing sexual relations, the generation of the human person is objectively deprived of its proper perfection: namely, that of being the result and fruit of a conjugal act in which the spouses can become 'cooperators with God for giving life to a new person.[114]

---

111 Ibid., II, B/4, a. (The emphasis is added); the citation refers to Pius XII, *Discourse to Those Taking Part in the Second World Congress on Fertility and Sterility*.
112 *Donum Vitae*, II, B/4, a.
113 Ibid., II, B/4, c.
114 Ibid., II, B/5. The internal quotation is taken from *Familiaris Consortio*, n. 14.

Indeed, the desire to have a child through in vitro fertilization is judged by the Instruction to be equivalent to treating the child as a product owing to the technical manipulations and decisions of both the spouses and the medical professionals apart from the process itself which has its own meaning of productivity. All of this is "incompatible with the equality of personal dignity between the child and those who give him life"[115]; this gives an impression of injustice to the child.

Thirdly, the document indicates that based on the "language of the body," the simple case cannot be morally licit because it is a mode of generation of life which fails to acknowledge the deep and intrinsic human significance of the personal gift, bodily and spiritual in nature of husband and wife to one another in the marital act.[116] The Instruction therefore declares:

> In order to respect the language of their bodies and their natural generosity, the conjugal union must take place with respect for its openness to procreation; and the procreation of a person must be the fruit and result of married love. The origin of the human being thus follows from a procreation that is 'linked to the union, not only biological but also spiritual, of the parents, made one by the bond of marriage.' Fertilization achieved outside the bodies of the couple remains by this very fact deprived of the meanings and values which are expressed in the language of the body and in the union of the persons.[117]

It is in accordance to the language of the body that couples mutually express their self-gift to each other in complete and total manner reaching its peak in the conjugal act. This act of self-gift is motivated by the "spousal meanings" of the body, which includes the parental ones. The entire act since it pertains to the human person, involves the couple's corporal and spiritual dimensions; it is in "their bodies and through their bodies that the spouses consummate their marriage and able to become father and mother."[118] It appears that the centrality of the Instruction's argument against the simple case lies in the fact that fertilization is brought about outside the specific act of the conjugal sexual union.

---

115 May, *Marriage*, 80.
116 Ibid., 81.
117 *Donum Vitae*, II, B/ 4, b.
118 Ibid.

Finally, the document acknowledges that although the simple case may not be complicated with the compromise of abortive practice of destroying embryos and with masturbation, it remains yet a technique that is morally illicit because it deprives human procreation of the dignity, which is proper and connatural to it. According to the Instruction,

> Certainly, homologous IVF and ET fertilization is not marked by all that ethical negativity found in extra-conjugal procreation; the family and marriage continue to constitute the setting for the birth and upbringing of children. Nevertheless, ... the Church remains opposed from the moral point of view to 'in vitro' fertilization. Such fertilization is in itself illicit and in opposition to the dignity of procreation of the conjugal union, even when everything is done to avoid the death of human embryo.[119]

In summary, it can be discerned from the document's evaluation regarding the simple case, that marriage inasmuch as it remains the context for the generation of human life, is not sufficient to make the simple case morally licit. This is so, because it is profoundly a moral question to separate procreation from the sexual act. In fact, it is the very reason why the simple case is judged to be morally wrong. The good intention of the couple to have a child cannot make up for the immorality of achieving the desire outside the specific act of their marital act.

There is a relationship between the simple case IVF-ET and homologous artificial insemination based on the fact that both methods are between husband and wife. However, each one requires a specific moral evaluation because the mode of achieving fertilization is different. While the Instruction condemns unambiguously the simple case IVF-ET, certain procedures of homologous artificial insemination have been left open without a definite judgment on their acceptability or otherwise. *Donum Vitae*'s position on these methods of human artificial follows the teaching of Pius XII who did not foreclose *a priori* every method of homologous artificial insemination on the basis that they are artificial. The basic moral or ethical evaluation of these procedures is related to the goal for which they are sought within marriage and the methods used as well as the techniques involved for their application. In the absence of a definite judgment, it is required as Ratzinger indicated, that the Catholic doctors are encouraged

---

119 Ibid., II, B/5.

to rely on their informed conscience in their decision on either to perform these techniques or not.[120] The classic theological principles and concrete circumstances would be useful to the doctor's decision, and this means that the Catholic doctors would need to stay tuned to current Catholic theological and ethical developments. In fact, this apparent silence of the Magisterium regarding its stance on these procedures has generated series of debates on the acceptability of these methods, whether they truly assist the conjugal act or they substitute for it.

On account of this, some ethicists and moral theologians have suggested that the technique of homologous artificial insemination can be classified into two types, namely, homologous artificial insemination *properly speaking* (this procedure replaces the conjugal act) and artificial insemination *improperly speaking* (this procedure is believed to assist the conjugal act).[121] There are particular techniques of homologous artificial insemination which theologians believe can assist the conjugal act to achieve its goal of procreation and these belong to the homologous artificial insemination *improperly speaking*. These procedures include Gamete IntraFallopian Transfer (GIFT), Low Tubal Ovum Transfer (LTOT) and Tubal Ovum Transfer with Sperm (TOTS). It may be pertinent to underscore that the term "artificial" as used in the distinction on artificial insemination or for artificial procreation is not immoral in itself. But, it can be immoral if it replaces the conjugal act and so be considered unnatural to the procreative process. On the other hand, when it does not replace the conjugal act but assists it, it is not unnatural but rational and morally licit. From an ethical viewpoint, this distinction can help to differentiate between the technique that is properly an assisted procreative technology from that which is a replacement or substitution to

---

120 Cf. The National Catholic News Service, "Instruction on Respect for Human Life in Its Origin and on the Dignity of Procreation," in *Origins* 16, 40 (1987): Marginal note, 699.

121 Sgreccia, *Personalist Bioethics*, 482; Ángel Rodríguez-Luño, *Scelti in Cristo per Essere Santi*, Vol. 3 (Edusc, Roma, 2008), 216. For a profound study, the cited authors have offered an elaborate treatment of these procedures of artificial procreation considered to have the possibility of meeting the ethical requirement for a medical assistance to the conjugal act. The arguments regarding these procedures are deeply developed in this work because the principal procedure under consideration is the simple case and these open procedures.

the marital act. It is clear that the Instruction makes no judgment or specific reference to any of these techniques of homologous artificial insemination *improperly speaking*, but some Catholic theologians speculate on these procedures to include those we have mentioned, claiming that these techniques do not replace the conjugal act and so do not present moral difficulties like others. In his apparent support of these techniques of homologous artificial insemination *improperly speaking*, Sgreccia submits that:

> There are no contraindications for homologous artificial insemination, and it presents no moral difficulties so long as we are talking about therapeutic and holistic assistance to ensure that the conjugal act, which is complete in itself with all of its components (physical, psychological, and spiritual), can have a procreative result. This practice does not pose ethical problems even for the Magisterium of the Catholic Church, provided that the techniques applied [in particular for obtaining the semen] are moral in themselves. The semen can also be licitly treated to improve capacitation once it has been obtained.[122]

Our main preoccupation in this study is not on these methods of homologous insemination but the simple case IVF-ET. The few comments we have made on these open techniques could serve to clarify the distinction between the medical techniques that constitute assistance to the conjugal act and those that replace the conjugal act by which reason they are judged to be illicit by the Catholic Magisterium.

1.2.6. Relationship between Moral and Civil Law

The Instruction in this section invites political authorities and the legislators to intervene and formulate laws that would regulate the application of the emerging technological possibilities in the field of biomedicine. The Church is worried that if leaders of the civil government did not make haste to use its authority wisely to defend the fundamental values concerning the condition and integral vocation of the human person, the family and the institution of marriage which are constitutive elements of the society, the society could be heading towards self destruction by the handiwork of man. Since the state has the role to protect and promote the common good of all, its legislations must be shaped by moral law to enforce morality in the field of biomedical science and technology.

---

122 Sgreccia, *Personalist Bioethics*, 485.

Donum Vitae maintains that the human society is founded upon the institution of marriage that is an essential element in fostering the common good. And that the protection of life is the primary function of the political society, this role must be assumed without bias and discrimination on the quality of life since every human life enjoys the same rights and dignity as a gift from God. According to the Instruction, among the fundamental rights of the human person derived from natural law, two fundamental rights that are not concession from the civil society but which every human life is imbued with are: (a) the right to life and physical integrity from the moment of conception until death; and (b) the rights of the family and of marriage as an institution and, in this area, the child's right to be conceived, brought into the world and brought up by his parents. The document notes that if the state fails to recognize and protect the rights and lives of her citizens, especially the most vulnerable of them including the yet unborn precisely those at the embryonic stage, the foundation of her laws would be undermined.[123] The political authorities are therefore urged to make available their services in favor of everyone and of the family by legislating against the manipulation of the human subjects in whatever stage of development by harmful biomedical procedures.

Similarly, *Donum Vitae* sounds critical of the civil governments that it is beyond the competence of the political authorities to approve techniques of artificial procreation that replace what is properly inherent in spousal communion. It reminds Political authorities that they cannot give approval to the calling of a human being into existence through procedures that are detrimental to the child, parents and the holy union of matrimony. Therefore, the state is encouraged to avoid approving harmful methods of artificial procreation and to penalize those who engage in anti-human and anti-family procedures of which the simple case IVF is an example irrespective of it being less complicated morally than other similar procedures; techniques involving donation of gametes between persons who are not married, including post-mortem insemination, embryo banks, and surrogacy. Similarly, Ratzinger makes a strong case in his letter to Marcello Pera as the then president of the Italian Senate regarding the problems of

---

123 Ibid., III.

artificial procreation in connection with civil legislation. He feels that the problems inherent in artificial conception could be compelling to go too far. He explains that in the light of *Donum Vitae*, based on anthropological argument, while rejecting homologous fertilization extracorporeal as well as that of heterologous, it does not require the legislature to prohibit homologous conception extracorporeal. However, it would prefer that the legislature prohibits heterologous artificial fertilization by law, otherwise, it would renounce or undermine the values that are still protected by law in marriage.[124] This implies that while the state can be encouraged to make laws forbidding heterologous artificial procreation, it would be going to far beyond its jurisdiction to proscribe by law homologous artificial procreation. From the perspective of the Magisterium as indicated in *Donum Vitae*, it is not every form of homologous artificial fertilization that is morally illicit, especially those procedures that do not substitute or replace the conjugal act. The basis of this position just stated is both moral as well as anthropological. This consideration lies outside the sphere of the state legislation. In general, the rejection of human extracorporeal fertilization accords with common sense and rationality. Equally, the obligation to protect the values of marriage by the Church and the State requires it because of its inherent complications and problems pertaining to the values of human life and those of marriage.

Synthesis of the Chapter

In order to understand better the current debate on the simple case of homologous IVF-ET based on the magisterial teaching in *Donum Vitae*, this first chapter has undertaken a brief overview study from *Casti Connubii* to *Donum Vitae* concerning medical interventions in human procreation.

---

124 Joseph Ratzinger, "Lettera a Marcello Pera," in Marcello Pera and Joseph Ratzinger (eds.), *Senza Radici: Europa, Relativismo, Cristianesimo, Islam* (Milano: Arnoldo Mondatori Editrice, 2004), 120. "… la *Donum vitae*, pur rifiutando, sulla base di un'etica che argomenta antropologicamente, la fecondazione omologa come anche quella eterologa, non esige dal legislatore il divieto della fecondazione omologa extracorporea, ma vorrebbe comunque vedere esclusa la fecondazione eterologa anche per legge, in quanto altrimenti si rinuncerebbe al valore, ancora protetto per legge, del matrimonio."

In the light of these periods and magisterial teachings under review, there is a sign of gradual development and continuity of doctrine on the question of intervention in human procreation. In *Casti Connubii*, relying on the natural moral law and the Divine law, Pius XI expressed the truth that could be discerned for an argument concerning human procreation but his teaching seemed to address this question only indirectly, the seminal deposit of his doctrine on artificial fertilization cannot be refuted. Basically, he stressed that every marital act by necessity had to retain its intrinsic relationship with the transmission of life. After him, Pius XII who explicitly set the principle of inseparability of the conjugal act, using it to reject as illicit both artificial insemination and human in vitro fertilization that are achieved outside the marital act. He taught that the unitive and the procreative meanings of the conjugal act should not be positively separated within marriage for selfish reasons or vitiated by certain means. In formulating this principle, he left open for future study whether an unspecified procedure that simply assisted the conjugal act to achieve procreation without replacing it was licit. Further development on this doctrine is seen in the teaching of Paul VI in *Humanae Vitae*. In this document, the Pope affirmed and gave an insightful and elaborate formulation of the connection between the unitive and procreative aspects of the conjugal act. In relying on the articulations of previous magisterial documents on marriage and sexuality and more specifically on the conjugal act, Paul VI brought in the notion of "meaning" to the two aspects of the conjugal act, a development that was a novelty and foundational in a certain sense. In *Humanae Vitae*, we find a renewed significance of the Church's teaching on marriage and more specifically on the conjugal act seen as a human act of love. This doctrine was principally established against contraception but had implications for artificial procreation as well. In his turn, John XXIII directly criticized the procedures of artificial procreation. In *Mater et Magistra*, he taught that the transmission of human life is entrusted by nature to a personal and conscious act subject to the Divine laws and as such limited to marriage. Consequently, those techniques that may be licit for use in the reproduction of plants and animals cannot be used for man. For him, the dignity of man and the Divine laws do not admit of such means.

Indeed, in continuity and conformity to the different magisterial teachings regarding interventions in human procreation, the Vatican Instruction

Donum Vitae affirms and expounds on the basic general Catholic moral principles that regulate artificial procreation. First, the doctrine of inseparability of the two meanings of conjugal union and procreation intrinsically connected in the conjugal act is reiterated. Besides this principle of inseparability, the Instruction highlights, in a remarkable way, the principle of the unity of the human person as a unique being of body and soul expressed in the "language of the body" by the spouses. It is the fact of this spousal significance of the body that openness to new life is required. Another principle established in *Donum Vitae* is that human life is gift. It reveals that human life must be begotten as the fruit of mutual self-giving of the spouses in love and not produced *in vitro* as a product of technology. In fact, the Instruction *Donum Vitae* is reckoned as one significant compendium of the Church's teaching on the limits of interventions in human procreation and respect for human life in its origin. These basic principles used by the Magisterium are anthropologically and theologically derived. No doubts, the arguments employed by the Magisterium are also philosophically and ethically structured. It can simply be said that *Donum Vitae* bears the fruits of the application of the integral Church's true vision of man in relation to certain bioethical questions of the day.

In fact, as pertains to the simple case of homologous IVF-ET, the Magisterium considers it less problematic yet illicit. Based on the Church's teaching, the most fundamental and straightforward principle valid for the rejection of the simple case IVF-ET is the doctrine on inseparability of the two meanings of the conjugal act. However, other principles can equally be applied in tandem with this basic principle of inseparability. But for the dissenting theological opinion, it can be argued, that if it depended on this single principle as it appears, one cannot use this principle to rule out the moral acceptability of the simple case since it is not self-evident in this principle that procreation should not be achieved outside the conjugal act. At best, this principle requires that when the conjugal act is performed, the unitive and the procreative dimensions should be kept intact not that procreation should not occur outside the conjugal act. Besides this critical view, there exist other dissenting views against the teaching of *Donum Vitae* on the simple. It is the dissenting theological opinion that we now turn to in the next chapter.

Chapter Two Moral-Theological Arguments in Favor of the Simple Case of Homologous IVF-ET

Introduction

One of the objectives of our research is to examine some basic theological arguments in Catholic discourses on the simple case IVF-ET in the light of *Donum Vitae*. In this chapter we are concerned with the dissenting theological opinions against the Catholic magisterial conclusion on this procedure of artificial conception as expressed in the Instruction and in its update *Dignitas Personae*.[125] The dissenting views need attention and evaluation, not so much as to change the Church's doctrinal position but to widen the horizon of knowledge of the problem and as well as an opportunity to attempt a clearer exposition of the Catholic moral doctrine by means of other theological insights from some theologians. Our attempt here is more or less being attentive to the theological and scholarly reactions/contributions in response to the Instruction's invitation. While the document considers all forms of procreation by IVF and similar methods of fertilization outside the sexual intercourse to be inherently illicit, these authors differ in some aspects that deserve attention. It seems that the justification of the Church's position or the rejection of it demands an anthropological and ethical analysis and this cannot be found exclusively in *Donum Vitae* or *Dignitas Personae*; and as Martin Rhonheimer would indicate, these documents are instructions and not a treatise of moral theology: "An encyclical is intended to present the teaching of the Church, and as such to be a source for theological work, without itself performing that work; its authority does not consist in arguments, but rather in the apostolic authority of the Magisterium."[126]

---

125 Congregation for the Doctrine of the Faith, *Instruction Dignitas Personae on Certain Bioethical Questions and the Dignity of the Person*, 20 June 2008: AAS 100 (2008): 858–887.
126 Here, Rhonheimer reflects critically on the famous citation from *Humanae Vitae*, that there is an "inseparable connection willed by God and incapable of being broken by man on his own initiative, between the two meanings of the conjugal act, the unitive meaning and the procreative meaning." For

Indeed, it is with the same understanding that we undertake this inquiry to see why critics of the Instruction do what they do and to examine the strength, validity and weakness of their arguments. The moral stance of the Catholic Magisterium in *Donum Vitae* has received varied critical views. Proponents of these views seem to agree that the document has a fairly developed and clear teaching on the question of artificial procreation, the sources of its teaching stretching beyond the sphere of Christian religion. But this teaching lacks credibility because of its problematic understanding and application of natural law sexuality and procreation. For them, the teaching is overly physicalistic or biological in its development of norms, and this narrowness of interpretation impedes a constructive and persuasive evaluation of the simple case IVF-ET procedure.

Undoubtedly, the arguments by these moral theologians against *Donum Vitae* on the simple case IVF-ET extend beyond the real question of the issue in itself to the consultation process, preparation and methodology of the document. Critiques seem to reason that the weakness or limitations in its preparation have also affected its negative conclusion on the simple case. These authors accuse the Magisterium among other things of poor consultation network; that it was selective and secretive, that it avoided some

---

Rhonheimer, the claim that this corresponds to the will of God must be justified by way of an anthropological and ethical analysis. The realization of this cannot be found in the document of *Humanae Vitae* because it is an encyclical and not a treatise of moral theology. In other words, the Magisterium points out the direction but the moral theologians have the duty of working out the details by a rigorous argumentation proposed by the Magisterium. This view of Rhonheimer holds true in the current document. Bruno Schüller finds favor with Rhonheimer's position but their conclusions are different. Schüller agrees that the encyclical would be a moral exhortation and not a treatise of moral theology. But, he also adds that the encyclical as a moral instruction can equally give answers to serious moral questions through rigorous moral reasoning but he doubts if such answers have been presented as the result of rigorous moral reasoning in *Donum Vitae*. See Martin Rhonheimer, Natural Law and Practical Reason: A Thomist View of Moral Autonomy, English translation from the German by Gerald Malsbary (Fordham University Press, 2000), nn380–381; Bruno Schüller, "Paraenesis and Moral Argument in *Donum Vitae*," in Edmund D. Pellegrino (ed. et al.), *Gift of Life: Catholic Scholars Respond to the Vatican Instruction* (Washington, D.C.: Georgetown University Press, 1990), 81–98.

professionals who might hold contrary views from the preconceived conclusion of the Vatican. They also think that undue appeal to authority rather than professionals or scientific data characterizes the document. Other more fundamental issues raised center on the alleged misinterpretation of the natural moral law, the nature of the human person, improper understanding of infertility technology, lack of sympathy for the childless couples, inadequate interpretation of the conjugal act, unsubstantiated claims of indignity of the child by the simple case IVF-ET. It is worthy of note that the Magisterium has unequivocally stated that the rejection of the simple case IVF and some other ARTs is not on the grounds that science or technology is evil or is it based on the distinction between being *natural* or *artificial* but basically on the grounds of either assistance to the conjugal act or a replacement/substitution of the conjugal act. The following lines of evaluation of the thoughts of the critics would struggle to render the argument of the Instruction unconvincing, unjustifiable, ambiguous, misleading and theologically bereft of current realities. Among Catholic theologians maintaining a dissenting view against the Instruction's conclusion on the simple case IVF-ET is McCormick. It is remarkable that while he has not explicitly dedicated a particular work to argue in favor of the simple case, he has in many of his works committed himself to expressing his opposition to the Instruction's conclusion on this procedure. The major arguments advanced in this section of our work are basic areas that McCormick focuses his critique of the Instruction as well as expresses his support for the simple case. The subdivisions are furnished by the collation of the different dissenting views of Catholic scholars in general.

A. The Critique of *Donum Vitae*

1.1. An Overview of Its Argumentation against the Instruction

The Editorial of *America* of 1987 published shortly after the release of the Instruction *Donum Vitae*, had this impression:

> The document will be criticized as deductive in its method. Before pronouncing in vitro fertilization illicit even for married couples, the document says that first a question of principle must be clarified. ... 'look, before we begin this discussion, let's get one thing straight.' And by the time the discussion is over, it is clear that the initial principle (of limiting procreation to the sexual act which excludes the

use of in vitro fertilization) has, in fact ruled out beforehand the possibility of in vitro fertilization for married couples.[127]

It seems that the cited remarks capture what dissenters think count for one of the weaknesses of the document or rather, one reason why it is difficult to be accepted, that is, the alleged deductive methodology. An argument is said to be deductive when the truth of the conclusion depends on the truth of the premises. Here, there is no allowance for probability and future changes.[128] The document forecloses any possibility that the simple case IVF could be licit in any situation, this definitive conclusion informs the Editorials' position that the Instruction is deductive in its argumentation.

Again, the arguments against the document on the simple case IVF-ET extend beyond the real question of the simple case to the methodology of the consultation process in the drafting of the document. Critics seem to reason that the limitations in its preparation have also affected its negative conclusion on the simple case. These authors accuse the document of poor method of consultation. They also think that undue appeal to authority rather than professionals or scientific data characterizes the document. These preliminary views form the first bloc of the critique against the negative judgment of the Magisterium on the simple case IVF-ET. Other blocs of the critique are claims on the principle of totality, suggesting that the whole marital relationship is a conjugal act; that the moral object defining the simple case IVF-ET is in the intention to have a child and not the side effects of the procedure. The claim that the simple case is life enhancing, a

---

127 George W. Hunt, "New Vatican Instruction on Human Life and Procreation," in *America* 156, 12 (1987): 245. The emphasis is not original to the article but that of the researcher.

128 This point can be expressed also by saying that, in a deductive argument, the premises are intended to provide such strong support for the conclusion that, if the premises are true, then it would be *impossible* for the conclusion to be false. A deductive argument is either valid or not valid, that is all. In the contrary, an inductive argument or reasoning implies that logical process in which the conclusion proposed contains more information than the observations or experience on which it is based. The truth of the conclusion is verifiable only in terms of future experience and certainty is attainable only if all possible instances have been examined. Unlike the deductive argument, an inductive argument depends on probability.

kind of pro-life procedure and not endangering or contemptuous of new life as attested to in *Donum Vitae* is also central to the critique against the magisterial conclusion. The dissenting opinion has challenged the judgment that because the simple case is an imperfect act *ipso facto* an immoral means of procreation. In this first section will be treated the first bloc of the claims by the dissenting theological opinions against the Vatican Instruction *Donum Vitae* on the simple case IVF-ET.

1.2. Narrowness in Its Range of Consultation

It is in line with the tradition of the Catholic Magisterium to seek consultations with professionals from relevant fields in the preparation of any document that addresses issues that touch particular aspects of human life, aspects that require current scientific facts. Such was the case with *Donum Vitae*. In the Press conference given by Ratzinger, the then President of the Congregation for the Doctrine of the Faith, before the release of the document, he intimated that a wide scope of consultation was covered in the preparation of the Instruction. He indicated that many bishops across the globe were consulted including 62 moral theologians, 22 professionals among them were geneticists, physiologists, physicians, biologists from different nationalities and persuasions. This goes to confirm that the document was "the fruit of a vast consultation."[129] In contrast to this claim, some critics of *Donum Vitae* allege that the value of the document is far from being a work of adequate consultation. Theologians like McCormick, Harvey, Tauer and Vacek argue that the Instruction lacks basic and essential scientific and professional data, an indication that the consultation was carried out with bias.[130] For instance, Tauer reports that: "Many critics of

---

129 Cf. John Collins Harvey, "Speculations Regarding the History of *Donum Vitae*," in *Journal of Medicine and Philosophy* 14 (1989): 485. While the report of Ratzinger on the level consultation done in the course of preparing the document remains unconvincing to the dissenting theologians, in the course of our research we couldn't have access to confirm in the archives of the Congregation of the Doctrine of the Faith because such documents (contributions from those consulted) can only be released to the public after many years of the publication of the document in question.

130 Cf. Carol A. Tauer, "*Donum Vitae*: Dissenting Opinions on the "Simple Case" of In Vitro Fertilization," in *Philosophy and Medicine* 53 (1997): 125–146;

the process used by the Congregation for the Doctrine of the Faith (CDF) described its consultation process as secretive, narrow, restricted to those who held conservative position, purely clerical and male, non-ecumenical, and lacking in adequate scientific expertise."[131] These dissenting theologians insinuate that renowned professionals in IVF may not have been consulted. McCormick, for the sake of example alleges, that consultation was limited largely to Europe that is younger and not well experienced in the field of bioethics, in medical assisted procreation and neglected the United States of America that is a decade older in the field.[132]

In anticipation of the outcome of the magisterial pronouncements, or rather, before the Vatican finished the composition of the Instruction, McCormick had gone to write an article in the *America* detailing what he calls "unsolicited suggestions" that the Vatican could adopt as criteria in the composition of the document. He claims to have been informed "unofficially" that the document was being prepared. While proposing in one of the criteria that the Vatican could "adopt an open and processive procedural model," he laments that usually, the

> Vatican documents are conceived and drafted in almost investigative secrecy. The slightest leak becomes a pontifical betrayal. Documents seem to appear from nowhere. Outsiders have no idea of the persons consulted, the drafters, the process. All we know is that they are 'official'. They invite and support the suspicion that there is something to hide, that consultation was selective according to predetermined position.[133]

McCormick's understanding of "open and processive procedural model," indicates almost the exact opposite of what he claims about the Church's documents above. He goes on to ask rhetorically, "Is the Holy See less active because a document goes through three or four public versions before

---

Richard A. McCormick, "The Vatican Document on Bioethics: Some Unsolicited Questions," in *America* 156 (1987a): 24–26; Edward V. Vacek, "Vatican Instruction on Reproductive Technology," in *Theological Studies* 49 (1988): 110–131; John C. Harvey, "Speculations Regarding the History of *Donum Vitae*," 481–491.

131 Tauer, "*Donum Vitae*: Dissenting Opinions on the "Simple Case" of In Vitro Fertilization," 130.
132 Ibid.
133 McCormick, "Some Unsolicited Questions," 26.

becoming final? Is the teaching less authoritative because it listens to all competences?"[134] While this article was published about two months before *Donum Vitae*, McCormick had anticipated its controversial nature at least to some of them who have always maintained contrary views knowing that it might not be anything different in the new document, this actually came to be the case. Shortly after its release, McCormick wrote:

> Neither the appearance nor the content of the Vatican's document, 'Instruction on Respect for Human Life in Its Origins and on the Dignity of Procreation: Replies to Certain Questions of the Day,' was a surprise... several Roman theologians close to the Holy See had publicly condemned even the 'simple case'... the sweeping condemnations of any reproductive technology that replaces sexual intercourse were hardly unexpected.[135]

In this quotation we can see those critics of the document, because they were not either consulted or their views considered contrary to those of the perceived drafters of the document, reasons were found to accuse the process of consultation of the Instruction or so it seems.

In fact, Harvey in his article titled: "Speculations on the History of *Donum Vitae*," aligns himself with some other theologians to criticize the origin of *Donum Vitae*. He speculates with some data and names of persons who participated in the drafting of the document. In his judgment, those involved were selected to meet the standard of the Vatican conservative ideology. He claims that:

> The possibility of a biased consultation is serious indeed. Monsignors Caffarra, Sgreccia, and Schooyans, Fathers Kieley and Serra, Professor William E. May are all known as conservative or classicist theologians. Only Fathers Cuyas and Ford are generally considered non-conservative but are hardly revisionists. Moreover, consultation with US experts in bioethics seems to have been indirect.[136]

With hindsight Harvey makes reference to McCormick's article published two months in view of *Donum Vitae,* that since the CDF is not specialized in bioethics it should consult widely on so serious and complex a subject. He went on to state:

---

134 Ibid.
135 Richard A. McCormick, "The Vatican Document on Bioethics: Two Responses," in *America* 156, 12 (1987): 247.
136 Harvey, "Speculations on the History of *Donum Vitae*," 490.

> One has to face the question whether consultation was obtained only from those individuals who would be known to support pre-established conclusions, such as Monsignor Carlo Caffarra, President of the Pontifical Institute for the Family, who had several times condemned In Vitro Fertilization for married couples (the simple case), rather than from theologians who disagreed with this position.[137]

For Harvey, "the consultants to whom CDF appears to have listened reflect only the conservative views favoured by the highest Vatican officials, not a consensus of Roman Catholic moral theologians worldwide."[138] In his turn, Vacek questions the seriousness of the consultation regarding *Donum Vitae* and asks whether potentially disagreeing voices were equally consulted. Vacek, like other critics on this point, doubts the claim of the Vatican officials that adequate consultation was done. For the critics, the references or bibliographical data in the document are obvious indications that the Magisterium failed to meet the required target. The critics' argument suggests that because of the alleged inadequacy in the consultation process, the Instruction's judgment to prohibit the simple case IVF-ET remains an error of judgment and theologically ambiguous.

From another perspective, critics feel that *Donum Vitae* appeals too much to the authority of past magisterial documents rather than to experience and current scientific realities. McCormick had written in his "Unsolicited Suggestions" that the contemporary tendency as a form of Catholic fundamentalism is frightening. What would he imply by this statement? His thoughts on this claim could be sipped or discerned from his submission as follows:

> [...] the contemporary tendency is, I am afraid, a form of Catholic fundamentalism – the idea that authority can substitute for or replace human experience, deliberation, grappling. It cannot. Therefore any document from the Holy See on bioethics must persuade. It cannot rely simply on formal authority to gain adherents. Indeed, the more the Church interventions appeal to their authority, the more they unwittingly underline their own weaknesses.[139]

---

137 Ibid.
138 Ibid.
139 McCormick, "Some Unsolicited Questions," 26; Schüller, "Paraenesis and Moral Argument," 98. Shüller feels that the argumentation in *Donum Vitae* depends almost entirely on the authority of the Magisterium rather than on the validity and strength of reasoning itself. He claims to share the submission of Hannah Arendt who had noted earlier that "Authority ... is incompatible

Furthermore, sequel to the release of *Donum Vitae*, McCormick felt disappointed that the document was a repetition of past limitations of making references only to the previous Church's documents. He indicates that the Instruction is bereft of current theological and scientific facts and insensitive to the need and plight of childless couples. He therefore claims that:

> The Pope must depend on theological advisors who, like all of us, are pilgrims and see only darkly. There are two points to emphasize in saying this. First, when teaching on doctrinal questions, the Pope must be careful to prevent his circle of advisors narrowing so as to exclude legitimate currents of theological thought, as Rahner has repeatedly noted. Second, even with the broadest consultation, authoritative teaching will unavoidably be time and culture-conditioned. A certain form of ecclesiastical fundamentalism tends to forget this.[140]

Similarly, to emphasize the supposed lack in *Donum Vitae*'s judgment on the simple case, Tauer in her essay observes:

> Internal evidence also indicates that research and consultation were narrow. Footnotes consist almost entirely of other pronouncements of the Magisterium. Theologians and bioethicists are not cited, although they have produced an enormous amount of writing on these topics. Similarly, the studies and recommendations of professional and government commissions on bioethics appear to be ignored.
>
> By early 1987 at least 85 major statements representing at least 25 different countries were available (Walters, 1987, p. 4). At that time LeRoy Walters developed a detailed analysis of fifteen of the most significant statements, mainly representing government commissions in the U.S., United Kingdom, Australia, France, Germany, Spain, and the Netherlands. These fifteen statements all agreed that homologous IVF was ethically acceptable (1987, pp. 5–7). The fact that *Donum Vitae* does not acknowledge that consensus weakens its credibility.
>
> While *Donum Vitae* is accurate in its references to scientific and medical procedures, it includes no documentation from those who are involved in the research and practice with these procedures. Perhaps more importantly, it lacks any concrete empirical data on the experience of married couples, whether parents or infertile. While it often refers to such experience, references are either abstractions or assumptions that are not validated.[141]

---

with persuasion which proposes equality and works through a process of argumentation. Where arguments are used, authority is left in abeyance." Cf. Hannah Arendt, *Between Past and Future* (Harmondsworth: Penguin Books, 1977), 93. Cited in Schüller, "Paraenesis and Moral Argument," 98.
140 McCormick, *Critical Thinking*, 340.
141 Tauer, "Dissenting Opinion on the Simple Case," 131.

Regarding the origin of *Donum Vitae*, we can conclude that critics accuse the CDF of poor or narrow consultation with relevant professionals, authoritative and fundamentalist in content and approach. They equally claim that the document fails to meet the current theological thought and experience in bioethics, indicating a significant lack of consensus among the believing community. Hence, the Instruction's conclusion on the simple case lacks credibility.

1.3. The Alleged Physicalism or Biologism of *Donum Vitae*

The basic debate here centers on the understanding of the anthropology that could be read in the Instruction. Dissenting opinion on the magisterial teaching on the simple case IVF claims that the moral norms in the *Donum Vitae* constitute a form of physicalism or biologism. The dissenting theologians deny that the anthropology used by the Magisterium is dualistic, not in conformity with the true nature of the couple as persons of bodily and spiritual dimensions. Despite the Instruction's assertion that its natural law cannot simply be a set of norms on the biological level, its critics insist that the conclusion of the Instruction does not affirm or justify its assertion. The document, regarding the moral criteria to adopt based on the anthropology of man, observes from the outset that:

> By virtue of its substantial union with a spiritual soul, the human body cannot be considered as a mere complex of tissues, organs and functions, nor can it be evaluated in the same way as the body of animals; rather it is a constitutive part of the person who manifests and expresses himself through it. The natural moral law expresses and lays down the purposes, rights and duties which are based upon the bodily and spiritual nature of the human person. Therefore this law cannot be thought of as simply a set of norms on the biological level; rather it must be defined as the rational order whereby man is called by the Creator to direct and regulate his life and actions and in particular to make use of his own body.[142]

McCormick, like others, argues that the idea of the magisterium suggesting that in every act of sexual act of sexual intercourse, the unitive and the procreative dimensions must be inseparable implies that every act of intercourse is in some sense procreative. He debunks this claim to be unrealistic. To substantiate his claim he poses a rhetorical question by asking, what

---

142 *Donum Vitae*, Introd., 3.

does it mean to attribute a procreative dimension to sexual union when it is known to be infertile (e.g., because of age)? For him, it is simply and in every respect a non-procreative act. Therefore he concludes:

> To maintain that such an action is 'open to procreation' and maintains the inseparability of the unitive-procreative dimensions make no sense. The action is unobstructed, to be sure. But to argue that it must (morally) be unobstructed is to attribute an overriding moral value to physical obstructedness. This is why many theologians see in this analysis a form of 'physicalism.'[143]

McCormick's view suggests that in emphasizing that every specific conjugal act must be considered procreative, the Instruction is overlooking one aspect of the human person, and that is precisely the spiritual. This for him is negative and improper and that is why its judgment on the simple case is negative. He argues that if the integrality of the couple as persons is to be considered, their bodily and spiritual dimensions are to be properly recognized, otherwise, we cannot say the human person must be brought into being as the fruit of the specific sexual act. The necessary connection between the conjugal act and procreation seems doubtful since experience shows that it is not always true that every sexual act results in procreation.

From another angle of alleged biologism of *Donum Vitae* is found what Todd A. Salzman and Michael E. Lawler identify as "a methodological shift" of argument, a kind of different criteria to evaluate the same problem and then arriving at the same conclusion. According to these authors, the Vatican seems to use a Personalist principle to evaluate heterologous artificial reproduction but in the case of homologous artificial reproduction, it shifts its emphasis to biological principle. They illustrate that:

> The CDF's treatment of AFH opens with the question: "What connection is required from the moral point of view between procreation and the conjugal act?' The shift in question from 'Dignity of the couple and the Truth of Marriage' to 'Procreation and the Conjugal Act' reflects a methodological shift from the primacy of a relational, personalist emphasis to the primacy of an act-centered, biological emphasis."[144]

---

143 McCormick, *Critical Calling*, 348.
144 Todd A. Salzman and Michael E. Lawler, *The Sexual Person: Toward a Renewed Catholic Anthropology* (Washington, D.C: Georgetown University Press, 2008), 244. The internal citation is from *Donum Vitae*, II, B/4.

Having stated this, Salzman and Lawler agree that the rejection of heterologous reproductive technologies seems reasonable on account of the reasons advanced by the Instruction.[145] What remains doubtful and unreasonable for these authors is the rejection of homologous artificial procreation that does not present the same relational complications like the ones involving a donor. Why the shift of argument from marital relationship in general to the inseparability principle in the contexts? For Salzman and Lawler,

> All that can be claimed with certainty in the case of AFH is that the act of sexual intercourse is not *immediately* responsible for procreation. This point, however, though it gives us insight into the procedure facilitating reproduction, gives us no insight into the *moral meaning* of that procedure… moral meaning is discerned not through the givenness of reality, in this case the *givenness* of the use of technology and science to assist reproduction, but in the *meaning* of those facts for human relationships. If the same personalist principle were to be applied to AFD, one could come to a different conclusion about the morality of AFH.[146]

With this submission, these authors believe that the Vatican's insistence on sexual intercourse as the only licit and acceptable means of procreation, and for the singular reason that the simple case of IVF is proscribed, makes its judgment biologically principled and *ipso facto* practically unrealistic.

In the research carried out by John Doerfler,[147] he identifies three elements which are present in the argument of the dissenting theologians: first, the human person adequately considered; second, the hierarchy of values; and third, the physical as instrument of the person. The categorization of these elements does not depend on the order of importance but on the logic of convenience.

1.3.1. Adequate Consideration of the Human Person

There is no doubting the fact that the nature of the human person embraces the physical, spiritual, emotional, social, rational, intellectual, volitional, biological but man can simply be defined as a being of bodily and spiritual

---

145 Ibid; *Donum Vitae*, II, A.
146 Salzman and Lawler, *The Sexual Person*, 245.
147 John Doerfler, *Donum Vitae Twenty Years After: The Debate whether it is Intrinsically Evil to Generate Human Life by Means other than the Marital Act* (Dissertation, Rome: Pontificia Universitas Lateranensis, Pontifiium Instittutum Joannes Paulus II, Studiorum Matrimonii et Familiae, 2010), 11–18.

composition. Some critics of *Donum Vitae* lay claim to these aspects of the human person in their argument in varied ways. Louis Janssens for instance claiming to rely on the teaching of *Gaudium et Spes*, develops eight attributes as dimensions of the human person upon which the integrity of the human person should be based to evaluate the morality of his actions. In other words, Janssens proposes that to determine the morality of an act, it is not sufficient to rely solely on the object or physical dimension of the act as the Magisterium frequently does in her evaluation of sexual and reproductive issues. For Janssens, the human person is (1) a subject, (2) in corporeality, (3) in relation to the material world, (4) in relation to others, (5) in relation to social groups, (6) in relation to God, (7) a developmental historical being, and (8) fundamentally equal to all human persons and yet uniquely original.[148] Janssens claims that his postulations agree with the personalism of *Gaudium et Spes* that calls for an adequate consideration of the human person in his dimensions in the evaluation of his acts. With this in mind, Janssens is critical at *Donum Vitae*'s rejection of the simple case IVF. Because, it seems to him that only the physical dimension of the conjugal act was considered by the Magisterium neglecting other dimensions that are equally constitutive of the human person. In other words, the human person was not integrally or adequately considered in *Donum Vitae*. Janssens hereby suggests that norms guiding sexual ethics should not always be posited on absolutes because of the existential contexts of human relationships.

Similar to Janssens' argument, Porter in her evaluation of the Vatican's Instruction concerning human procreation and specifically on the so-called simple case IVF, alleges that the principle of the document's judgment is not well grounded on the true nature of the person and of procreation. Referring to the principle of natural moral law of the Instruction, she argues: "this principle rests on a particular analysis of the structure and the intrinsic purposes of the sexual act. But of course, in the procedure of artificial procreation, there is no act of sexual intercourse going on, to be tampered with or violated."[149] Porter agrees with Janssens and McCormick

---

[148] Louis Janssens, "Artificial Insemination: Ethical Considerations," in *Louvain Studies* 8 (1980): 4.
[149] Porter, "Human Needs and Natural Law," 97.

among others to assert that the Instruction has a physicalist basis for the formation of moral norms. In this sense, the nature of the human person is inadequately considered. She claims that the natural, biological functions of the human organism have definite purposes, which can be recognized as such and which place moral parameters on human activity. Traditionally, the sexual function was seen within this framework as having only one primary purpose, namely, the procreation of children.[150] She seems to conclude that this method of moral reasoning does no justice to the correct evaluation of the nature of marriage and the generation of human life.

Furthermore, on the same point of inadequate consideration of the human nature, even before the release of *Donum Vitae*, McCormick who was privileged to get hold of news of its preparation, responded with an article hoping it might contribute to the content or methodology of the Instruction. In the article he raises some concerns on the Church's teaching on reproductive technologies, which he claims experience reveals it had always rested on some sort of physicalism or biologism. He therefore encouraged that the Vatican II's criterion for the moral wrongness or rightness should be taken seriously in the new document on bioethics. In the light of *Gaudium et Spes* number 51, he sustains that the moral judgment on the reproductive procedures must be based *on the nature of the person and his acts*. He argues that the italicized words in the sentence signify two things according to the official theological commentary. First, that the phrase presents a general criterion for judging moral right and wrong; that is, one that applies to all human activity, not just to the sexual sphere. And second, the human person refers to the person 'integrally and adequately considered.' With hindsight he states:

> For instance, in the past the criteriological significance of sexual conduct was found in its procreativity. Thus sexual intercourse was seen as 'the procreative act.' Deviations from this finality and significance were viewed as morally wrong and the decisive factor in judging conduct. The 'person integrally and adequately considered' goes beyond such biological givenness.[151]

All this goes to explain how the moral tradition of the Magisterium has been in history under the critique of dissenting theologians. In the same vein,

---

150 Ibid., 96.
151 McCormick, "Some Unsolicited Suggestions," 26.

The Critique of *Donum Vitae* 103

Thomas A. Shannon claims that essentially the argument of *Donum Vitae* has the same implications as that of *Humanae Vitae* that proscribes artificial contraception. In his allegation, he appeals to the authority of majority opinion and to Vatican II. He notes: "The majority of commentators, Catholic and non-Catholic alike, reject the primacy given to a biological structure over the personal dimension of the act of married intercourse. This overly biological reading of the natural law fits uneasily with the ethical standard suggested in the Vatican II document *Gaudium et Spes*."[152] Shannon continues,

> Many would argue that the key to moral analysis is whether marriage as a whole is open to procreation, not whether an individual act is. And even here, the tradition notes exceptions. Beginning with *Casti Connubii* and continuing through *Humanae Vitae*, valid reasons for avoiding conception (without the use of contraception of course) included the health of the mother and the need to care for the welfare and education of one's current family. And much earlier Thomas Aquinas noted that reproduction was an obligation that fell on the species, not on any particular individual.[153]

Having stated this, Shannon concludes that *Donum Vitae* deviates from this tradition and therein lies an irony in its moral analysis of the simple case. Shannon explains that within the context of marriage, two individuals are attempting to have a child. That is the object and intent of everything done within the context of artificial procreation. But, *Donum Vitae* focuses only on the physical integrity of the act of sexual intercourse and ignores 'the fact that husband and wife are seeking to become father and mother,' which of course is what the tradition says is the goal of marriage. He therefore claims: "Why the physical integrity of the act should take moral priority over the intention of the husband and wife to become mother and

---

152 Thomas A. Shannon, "Reproductive Technologies: Ethical and Religious Issues," in Thomas A. Shannon (ed.), *Reproductive Technologies: A Reader* (New York: A Sheed & Ward Book, 2004), 42. The suggestion from the document of Vatican II is from *Gaudium et Spes*, n. 51, which states that "… the moral aspects of any procedure does not depend solely on sincere intentions or on an evaluation of motives, but must be determined by objective standards. These, based on the nature of the human person and his acts, preserve the full sense of mutual self-giving and human procreation in the context of true love."
153 Ibid. (The emphasis is added).

father through the use of their own genetic material is both unexplained and unclear."[154] The insinuations expressed by Shannon like some other critics of *Donum Vitae*, that its argument on the simple case is misplaced, misapplied and inconsistent with Catholic tradition have rigorously been responded to in many other theological works which we shall treat in the next chapter.

Furthermore, in the book co-authored by Shannon and Cahill, one finds again an evidently vigorous critique of *Donum Vitae* on the alleged physicalist approach in the formulation and application of moral norms regarding the simple case. For instance, analyzing the Vatican's Instruction they observe that:

> Those norms prescribing the morality of sexual and procreative acts that are affirmed currently by the teaching authority of the Church, are the same norms that were originally derived from the more act-focused and often individualist understanding of sexuality... this often delineates human sexual 'nature in terms of physical nature (the integrity of the reproductive process), so that norms regarding sexuality are grounded primarily in that structure, rather than on the interpersonal meanings of sexual acts in relation to marital and parental love.[155]

They go further to assume that there is a less than adequate respect for the integrity of body and soul, in which both are valued together and together form an object of moral reflection. Once sexual morality is tied decisively to the physical components of sexual acts, it becomes difficult to make exceptions to the norms so derived, even to serve the personal good of the spouses, children, or families. In accusing the Magisterium of not considering adequately the nature of the person in his bodily and spiritual dimensions, these authors indicate that "moral inappropriateness is indicated at least in cases in which the ostensible justification of some 'purely biological' act is contingent on our ability to deny any significant connection at all of the person as a whole with that aspect of his or her biology which is to be involved."[156] Therefore, they believe that if dualism is a

---

154 Ibid. The internal quotation is an insight taken from James Keenan, "Moral Horizons in Health Care: Reproductive Technologies and Catholic Identity," in *Philosophy and Medicine* 53 (1997): 61–62.
155 Shannon and Cahill, *Religion and Artificial Procreation*, 51.
156 Ibid.

requisite maneuver in the justification of a 'biological' act, then both the justifying process and the act are suspects. By this claim, Cahill and Shannon are indicating that when only one aspect of the person is focused on, either on the body or on the spirit, the relevance of the other is disproportionately diminished and even evaluated in the negative light. This is similar to what other dissenting theologians have tried to point out, claiming that the Instruction by emphasizing the conjugal act as the specific and the only source of a child and by which the morality of artificial procreation must be based, tends to ignore the spiritual dimension of the whole person and of the procreative process. For them, this is incorrect because the conjugal act is one among many dimensions of the person and of human procreation.

1.3.2. Hierarchy of Values of the Human Person

Some proponents of the simple case IVF-ET argue that some human values are more important and higher than others. This reasoning has implications for the evaluation of the techniques of artificial procreation. This plays a role in the anthropological methodology of the dissenting theologians. Taken for granted that assisted procreative technologies should be evaluated based on the integral nature of the human person in his bodily and spiritual dimensions, critics push forward that beyond this criterion, hierarchy of human values is another significant factor for consideration. Following this school of thought, some dissenting theologians think that this aspect is apparently missing in *Donum Vitae*, otherwise the simple case IVF would not have merited a negative judgment. Proponents of this classification observe that marriage relationship as a whole or interpersonal relationship has priority over procreation. This suggests that the total relationship of the couple has a value in itself that is higher and by implication constitutes a more important criterion to situate procreation than on a particular physical act that is only an aspect in the entire marriage. For instance, Cahill writes that "I see no convincing argument that homologous techniques may not be evaluated as appropriate interventions in the presence of physical abnormalities, to accomplish the unity of love and procreation in the sexually expressed relation of a couple."[157] The only limits to procreative

---

157 Cahill, "What is the 'Nature' of the Unity of Sex, Love and Procreation? A Response to Elio Sgreccia," in *Gift of Life*, 147.

technologies in her views would be in a situation where either of the gametes comes from a third party, that is, heterologous artificial procreation. She claims that biological manipulation of either or both of the persons, who are already in marriage in order to achieve procreation, could be morally licit. The invasive nature of the procedure or the mediating role of the technology seems to be a neutral moral factor in her consideration. To explain her point, Cahill sustains that marriage relationship has three important values: love, sex and procreation; of these three values, the love relationship takes precedence. This is because, as she claims, it is a personal value while the other two are in the category of "physical goods and values."[158] And so, when *Donum Vitae* places emphasis instead on sexual intercourse, this cannot be a good moral judgment. By this, she accuses the document of setting moral principles that concern marriage and human procreation based on specific human actions rather than on marriage relationship that she claims to be more valuable. In this perspective, Cahill would argue that if biology sets the limits or basis for the morality of reproductive technologies, human freedom would be hampered. The proper and only limits that biology can set limit while respecting human freedom can be better understood this way:

> Biology sets a rightful limit only when a biological act or intervention entails an inappropriate involvement of the person whose 'biology' is in question. Thus biological manipulation of one (or both) of two persons already within a morally good relationship (marriage), in order to further a proper end of that relationship (procreation), is morally acceptable. It does not distort or change the basic personal relationship within which procreation is accomplished biologically: marriage. This remains true even if that accomplishment entails a biomedical replacement for sexual intercourse in the process of conception. The manipulation of reproductive biology still remains within the parameters of an appropriate and morally valid reproductive relationship of persons.[159]

The concern of Cahill suggests that marital relationship is the only legitimate factor that should empower the couples to seek for a child without any restriction and doing so through the simple case IVF is appropriate. While she insists that marriage relationship is the basic and most important

---

158 Ibid.,142.
159 Ibid., 143.

value in which the morality of reproductive technologies should be evaluated, the Instruction on its part indicates that the conjugal act, that personal sex act specific to the couple, ought to be the decisive factor for the moral evaluation of artificial procreation because human life owes its existence to it. In the contrary, for Cahill, "Physical goods and values can have an important relation to human relationships, but they are expressive and contributory, rather than fundamentally constitutive of such relationships."[160] In the light of this statement, Cahill considers the conjugal act not with the kind of importance the Instruction places on it. She thinks of the marital sexual act as merely a contributory, assisting act for procreation that is situated within the larger marital relationship. The positions of the Vatican and that of Cahill are at variance to each other. Both positions however agree that the sexual act of the couple is relevant for procreation. But, while *Donum Vitae* unequivocally emphasizes that procreation is ordained and should morally be a result of the specific sexual act of the couple, Cahill does not see the status of the marital sexual act as being the only act from which procreation should come. In other words, Cahill maintains the view that procreation can still be legitimate outside the specific sexual act of the couple but the totality of the existing sexual relations. Therefore, the simple case IVF is a legitimate means of procreation in her view.

Obviously, Shannon and Cahill are some of the scholars who strongly maintain that interpersonal love relationship of the spouses has a priority over and above the physical, procreative processes. This duo argues that to place the physical over the overall interpersonal relationship does not respect adequately the true nature of the human person in his body-soul unity. The claim that in its proper consideration, it can be sustained that

> Within the trinity of love, sex, and procreation, it is love that is fundamental, most humanly distinctive, and thus most morally important. Sex and procreation

---

160 Ibid., 142. Cahill responds to Sgreccia who argues that in IVF, 'procreation is not closely related to the act of conjugal love but the biologist's *technical activity*.' See Elio Sgreccia, "Moral Theology and Artificial Procreation in Light of *Donum Vitae*," in *Gift of Life*, 118; Lisa S. Cahill, *Sex, Gender, and Christian Ethics* (Cambridge: Cambridge University Press, 1996), 233; Ibid., "Catholic Sexual Ethics and the Dignity of the Person: A Double Message," in *Theological Studies* 50 (1989): 147; Louis Janssens, "Artificial Insemination: Ethical Consideration," in *Louvain Studies* 8 (1980): 4.

are not merely dispensable goods, but their moral meaning can be defined fully only within the interpersonal relationship of the persons who cooperate in realizing these goods.[161]

The spiritual and relational aspect of the human person according to Shannon and Cahill is most properly human and *ipso facto*, is of higher value than the sexual act. This suggests that the physical dimensions of the spouses in procreation are not properly personal, and, therefore, have lesser value.[162] The implication then becomes similar to what Doerfler considers the summary of the dissenting anthropological reasoning, namely, that "the formation of moral norms regarding reproductive technologies must acknowledge that the interpersonal love of the spouses has the highest value. Consequently, basing norms on merely the physical aspect of procreation bespeaks the type of physicalism evident in *Donum Vitae*."[163]

1.3.3. The Body as Instrument of the Human Person

In the Theology of the Body of John Paul II as evident in *Donum Vitae*, one finds that the human body is not a mere instrument of the person but a fundamental aspect of him upon which other human values depend.[164] The bodily dimension of the person is inseparable from the spiritual in the reality of his being. Contrary to this understanding, some of the dissenting theologians argue that the physical dimension of the person is merely instrumental to the person's being. How can the human person be thought of without his body? Are the matter and form of the human person separable in reality? It does seem that some critics of *Donum Vitae* who argue for the moral acceptability of the simple case IVF are maintaining this position. This suggests that the bodily/physical dimension is inferior to the spiritual that they consider to be the personal dimension of the human person. How can an embodied being be separated by way of emphasizing one dimension at the expense of the other? McCormick expresses this idea when he argues that the person integrally and adequately considered goes beyond such biological givenness upon which the Magisterium sets its criteria of moral

---

161 Shannon and Cahill, *Religion and Artificial Procreation*, 53.
162 Doerfler, *Donum Vitae Twenty Years After*, 15.
163 Ibid.
164 Cf. *Donum Vitae*, Intro., 4.

evaluation.[165] The idea conveyed by the use of "beyond" in McCormick's argument suggests a form of hyperpersonalism and a denial of the biological or at least making the biological submerged in the spiritual.[166]

The theological opinion which considers the human body in terms of instrumentality, is somehow suggestive that the physical dimension of man which they consider lower in value to the spiritual, could be sacrificed or utilized for the enhancement of the higher one, which is the spiritual or relational (personal value). No doubt, in their argument for an adequately derivation of moral norms about marriage and procreation, Shannon and Cahill claim to have a proper consideration of the bodily and spiritual dimensions of human nature. But, unfortunately, while they criticize the Magisterium for act-centered sexual morality, they fall headlong into subjugating the body into the spiritual goods of man in such a way that only the spiritual becomes a criterion of moral judgment. In a separate article by Cahill on the Vatican's Instruction, she gives an impression of how the body could be used as a means to an end to achieve the person's higher values. She seems to suggest that the spiritual qualities or aspects of the person are more essential about the person than the physical. The likely conclusion to be drawn from her view is that the physical aspect of the person including his sexuality is inferior to the spiritual as far as the identity of the person or value of the person as a whole is concerned. For example, she observes that:

> "... about human nature in general and marriage in particular, is that while both the material and spiritual dimensions are essentially human and should play a normative role in understanding moral obligations, it is the spiritual (i.e., intellectual, affective, and volitional) characteristics which are distinctive of humanity, which are more important in our appreciation of all that human 'dignity' entails, and which thus deserve more protection in cases of moral conflict."[167]

---

165 McCormick, "Some Unsolicited Suggestions," 26.
166 Cf. Edward V. Vacek, "Notes on Moral Theology," in *Theological Studies* 49 (1988): 113–131, at 119.
167 Cahill, "Moral Traditions, Ethical Language," 514. It is worthy of note that there exists a grave concern on the problem of "ethical dualism" in bioethical discourses. Johnstone has written an article on this, identifying two forms of ethical dualism. First, the "physical dualism," which tends to elevate the physical aspects of man at the expense of the spiritual. The second, which is "instrumental dualism," promotes the spirit or mind and devalues the body. It is interesting to see that while the dissenting views criticize the Vatican

Considering her statement critically, one can say, Cahill is advocating that the physical aspects of the person are non-essential in the derivation of moral norms about human sexuality and about human procreation. She agrees that marriage and sexuality have the dimensions of spousal union and parenthood. But, in the circumstances where nature does not permit the couple to beget a child naturally, by the fact, that their spousal union is of primary relevance being categorized as spiritual and so they may achieve the secondary value of their union, the child through technological means. What is paramount in her reasoning is the marital relationship. She does not consider the means of procreation as a problem inasmuch as the value of the child is secondary to the marital union. This position could be found in the thoughts of Janssens as well. For him, interpersonal relationship is the ultimate criterion for the moral legitimacy prior to the value of corporeality in the decision for artificial procreation.[168]

The idea of subjecting the body under the spirit or better said, reducing the bodily dimensions of the spouses and by implication, procreation to serve the spiritual dimensions of love relations and other spiritual values are also expressed approvingly by Sidney Callahan, Vacek, Selling among others. Vacek for instance makes reference to Callahan indicating that in setting moral norms for artificial procreation, "the 'couple's life,' not procreation, should be foundational and primary."[169] The implication of this conclusion suggests that the "couple's life" which is their relationship takes

---

Instruction for being "physicalist," even though this charge is being debunked, one notices a similar pitfall when the same dissenting theologians like Cahill would elevate the spiritual values of the person to the detriment of the physical dimensions in such a way that the body becomes a mere instrument to realize the total value of the person. Cf. Brian V. Johnstone, "In Vitro Fertilization and Ethical Dualism," in The *Linacre Quarterly* 53 (1986): 66–79. See also Nicholas Tonti-Filippini, "Bioethics and Ethical Dualism," in *Linacre Quarterly* 54, 2 (1987): 77–80.

168 Cf. Salzman and Lawler, *The Sexual Person*, 104. Janssens unlike McCormick, Cahill and other dissenting Catholic theologians, suggests that artificial procreation involving a donor may be problematic but not illicit. His justification of artificial insemination by donor is generally considered by fellow dissents as an extreme position.

169 Vacek, "Notes on Moral Theology," 125; Sidney Callahan, "Lovemaking and Babymaking," in *Commonweal* 114 (1987): 237.

precedence over the procreative dimension of that interpersonal union. This is equally indicated by Selling's observation, that other values related to the person and marriage are more important than the physical ones. He argues that "The familial, social, historical, and transcendent values of procreating a unique yet equal human being may still be realized if the couple is capable of understanding their desire to achieve parenthood as an expression of their human, rather than merely their biological, potential."[170] For him, there are other resources connected to man like technology as the product of man's intelligence to achieve a new human life. It seems clear that these authors indicated above maintain the position that sees the human body as an instrument of the person serving only the interest of the spiritual dimension of the person.

1.4. Inadequate Use of Its Natural Law Methodology

The argument here is different from the one on alleged non-dualism of *Donum Vitae* as expressed by its critics. The argument in this section pertains to the application of the natural law theory. By natural law we understand man's participation in God's eternal law.[171] The Catholic Magisterium in evaluating the procedures of assisted reproductive technologies, in accordance with human anthropology, also makes use of criteria derived from natural law.[172] However, some of the critics of the Instruction concerning

---

170 Joseph A. Selling, "The Instruction on Respect for Life: II. Dealing with the Issues," in *Louvain Studies* 12 (1987): 330.
171 See *The Catechism of the Catholic Church* nn.1954–1955: "Man participates in the wisdom and goodness of the Creator who gives him mastery over his acts and the ability to govern himself with a view to the true and the good. The natural law expresses the original moral sense, which enables man to discern by reason the good and the evil, the truth and the lie [...]. The 'divine and moral' law shows man the way to follow so as to practice the good and attain his end. The natural law states the first and essential precepts which govern the moral life."
172 Cf. *Donum Vitae*, Introd., 3. "The natural moral law expresses and lays down the purposes, rights and duties which are based upon the bodily and spiritual nature of the human person. Therefore the law cannot be thought of as simply a set of norms on the biological level; rather it must be defined as the rational order whereby man is called by the Creator to direct and regulate his life and actions and in particular to make use of his own body."

artificial procreation have observed reservations on the document's methodology in the use of natural law theory. In the critiques of the Vatican's Instruction for condemning certain forms of procedures of artificial procreation including the simple case IVF, one prevalent argument rests on the natural law. Critics argue that the Church's derivation of the natural moral law is too physicalistic and a form of biologism. Cahill for instance attributes this failure to the Magisterium's interpretation of the natural law relying heavily on its own authority and not sufficiently on human experiences or reasonable consensus about basic human values. For this sake, the Church risks self-destruction as an effective moral teacher.[173] Her observation is prefixed on her earlier proposition that basically the basic assets of the natural law argument or interpretation depend on *objective moral order* and on the community of *moral discourse* it establishes.[174] Based on these factors, she claims, one cannot say that the Instruction *Donum Vitae* was properly formulated to reflect the natural law, as it should be. She goes further to argue that natural law demands dialogue among several sources because the understanding of values or natural moral law is not accessible to everyone easily. She feels that not even moral theology or the Magisterium possesses a timeless and precise set of moral rules regarding artificial reproduction in such a way as to translate in a language suitable to every epoch and in every situation. In the light of this, she avers:

> Moral understanding of values to be protected and rules specifying them can arise only out of an interaction among several sources: contemporary experience, including empirical science and medicine; the tradition of the Church, including the scripture, theology, and magisterium; and refined philosophical analysis, in which religious persons and teachers may cooperate with others in arriving at a better understanding of what the natural law demands in a particular area of moral practice.[175]

Secondly, Cahill believes that historical and cultural contextualization is absolutely crucial in order to communicate any moral message at all. She appeals to the thoughts of Joseph Fuchs thus:

---

173 Cahill, "The Unity of Sex, Love and Procreation," 144.
174 Ibid.
175 Ibid., 145.

> Revelation itself, and even more so tradition and the magisterium, already adhere to some theological assertions which are formulated as propositions. We should not forget, however, that these assertions are always necessarily formulated in the language of a particular horizon of thought, with its own way of posing questions. We have need not only of interpretation but also of a hermeneutic, in order correctly to translate into contemporary ways of questioning and understanding those things put differently in the sources of our faith and in the theology (theologies) of times past. Only in this way can we guarantee a genuine transmission of the content of our faith, and not just a verbal correctness which could produce a falsification or an inexact rendering of the tradition.[176]

She relies on this reference to Fuchs to support her argument, suggesting that the interpretation of the natural moral law is largely tied to time and circumstances. By implication, the authors of *Donum Vitae* in proscribing the simple case, failed to be current in light of contemporary experience and circumstances of married couples that are infertile. Hence, she claims to "... see no convincing argument that homologous techniques may not be evaluated as appropriate interventions in the presence of physical abnormalities, to accomplish the unity of love and procreation in the sexually expressed relation of a couple."[177]

Furthermore, some critics accuse the Magisterium of being a victim of naturalistic fallacy by deducing moral norms from biological data. Shannon for instance has no doubt that just like *Humanae Vitae* that was premised on the natural law but wrongly applied, so also is *Donum Vitae*. Both documents use the same argument but in a reverse way to proscribe contraception and artificial conception. For Shannon, the Magisterium in both documents betrays the right application of the natural law by prioritizing the biological processes and procedures in the understanding of the morality of sexual acts and of procreation.[178] He argues that such an interpretation portents a rejection or at least diminishing consequences of the moral significance of the couples' intention to behold the fruit of their marital union. He therefore feels that the goal of a family is "held hostage to biology" in the tradition that sees marriage as a family. Furthermore, he claims that:

---

176 Ibid. Cahill alludes to: Joseph Fuchs, *Personal Responsibility and Christian Morality* (Washington, D.C.: Georgetown University Press, 1983), 6.
177 Cahill, "The Unity of Sex, Love and Procreation," 147.
178 Shannon, "Reproductive Technologies," 46.

> ... moral integrity consists in discovering the metaphysical order embedded in the biological order and then conforming ourselves to both. Thus not only does the natural law perspective as represented here call for caution and a sense of limits but also mandates a genuine non-intervention in the biological order. This overly biological view of natural law in turn shapes the Roman Catholic understanding of marriage. The primary focus is on the physical integrity of sexual relations between the couple, rather than how a couple, might achieve a family within the context of their marriage or how marriage might contribute to the social good.[179]

The submission of Shannon is a critique not only of *Donum Vitae* but of other past magisterial documents which have come under attacks from some theologians. The frequently common theological tension among Catholic theologians and ethicists that the present Instruction is not spared focuses on whether to define the object of morality as one's intentions or the physical object. There is another dimension as to whether impersonal structures take precedent over the personal acts? And yet another: can the goal of a family, which is a major element in the theology of marriage, be frustrated because of malfunctioning biology? In fact, Shannon claims that the critics of the Instruction do recognize the significance of the physical dimension of the person, but are concerned about the obvious overemphasis placed on it in evaluating human acts. For Shannon, what critics do differently is to argue that the "the biological should not be understood as a physical process that is morally normative, but rather as the person's mode of presence in the world, a dynamic and developing reality, a body-self."[180] In the light of this, he claims human beings by this incarnational presence become present to and bound to the world, society, community, and the dynamic of history.

1.5. Summary

In the foregoing we presented some of the critiques centered on the methodology of the Instruction both in the process of composition and the application of moral norms. Firstly, critiques are drawn from the allegation of narrow consultation or rather selective consultation without adequate dialogue among contemporary experts from different divides. Secondly, the

---

179 Ibid., 47.
180 Ibid., 48.

Instruction is criticized for seemingly appealing to self-authority as seen in the document's profuse references to past magisterial documents rather than scientific and contemporary theories and experiences. Thirdly, the document's methodology of emphasizing that human procreation must be owed to the personal and specific sexual act of the couple is seen by critics to be an inadequate method of moral evaluation that depends on biological or physical acts for moral norms. The dissenting theological opinion would prefer that the decisive moral factor or act should be the whole marital relationship, the spiritual as a higher human value. Obviously, there are methodological differences between the Magisterium and the dissenting theologians, and the most central point of tension and disagreement revolves around the interpretation and application of the natural moral law. As in this section we have considered the issues on the document's methodology and preparation, the next section will center on the main issues in detail.

The main debate on the morality of the simple case IVF-ET and other means of human procreation revolves principally around the meaning of the conjugal act. There are indications that the dissenting theological opinion has a conception of what the conjugal act should be, different from what the Magisterium teaches and its defenders uphold. Since both the dissenting and the defending theological views belong to the circle of Catholic theological thoughts, we will briefly present what the Catholic doctrine teaches on the meaning of the conjugal act. This will precede the theological arguments that are critical of the Vatican Instruction for prohibiting the simple case IVF-ET with an appeal to the conjugal act.

B. On the Conjugal Act and Its Understanding by the Dissenting Theologians

1.1. An Overview

What is the conjugal act? The conjugal act is understood simply as the sexual intercourse or relationship between married spouses of different sex.[181] The conjugal act is also described as that distinctive personal gesture

---

[181] Selling has criticized the use of the concept "conjugal act" by the Magisterium. He understands this term as being synonymous with marital sexual intercourse. He refers to this term as used by the Magisterium as "euphemism," accusing

by which husband and wife donate and receive each other as a symbol of their communion in love and for life. The conjugal act is a personal act through which the man and woman as husband and wife participate in the blessings of marriage. By its natural order, the conjugal act or marital act has two basic dimensions of unity and procreation. In *Donum Vitae*, the Magisterium teaches, "… by its intimate structure, the conjugal act, while most closely uniting husband and wife, capacitates them for the generation of new lives, according to laws inscribed in the very being of man and of woman."[182] As it pertains to the simple case IVF-ET, the central message of *Donum Vitae* is located in its consideration of the natural value and significance of the conjugal act. This Instruction asserts that "the moral relevance of the link between the meanings of the conjugal act and between the goods of marriage as well as the unity of the human being and the dignity of his origin, demand that the procreation of a human person be brought about as the fruit of the conjugal act specific to the love between spouses."[183] This moral criterion affirmed by the Magisterium is said to flow from the nature of the human person suggesting that the cause of his being must march with the means by which he is brought into being. That is why the document sees the simple case IVF as "… neither in fact achieved nor positively willed as the expression and fruit of a specific conjugal union. … even if it is considered in the context of '*de facto*' existing sexual relations, the generation of the human person is objectively deprived of its proper

---

it of being vague. He argues that at first sight it appears accurate but can be misleading to some people. For him, it gives the impression that marital union is synonymous with a sexual compact. He feels that contrary to what is suggested by the sense in which the Magisterium uses this concept, there are many other conjugal acts such as conjugal acts of trust, empathy, understanding, generosity, of which all may form a particular kind of friendship. He concludes that the conjugal act of sexual intercourse is only one among many possible acts of conjugal acts. His critical observation is meant to reject the restriction of procreation to only the conjugal act rather than within the marital relationship as a whole. Cf. Selling, "The Instruction on Respect for Life: II. Dealing with the Issues." 335.

182 *Donum Vitae*, II, B/4, a. The document makes reference to Paul VI's encyclical letter *Humanae Vitae*, n. 12.
183 *Donum Vitae*, II, B/4, c.

perfection: namely that of being the result and fruit of a conjugal act."[184] In all of this, the principle of inseparability of the conjugal act which holds true for both contraception and artificial procreation, remains the foundation upon which the above articulations depend. As Johnstone tries to explain, the conjugal act is that particular physical structure in which the goods of marriage (love union and procreation) are realized.[185] This means that love and procreation as goods of the spirit are embodied values through the physical structures of the human body.

1.2. On the Principle of Totality and the Conjugal Act

There are disagreements among theologians on the proper understanding and application of the concept of the principle of totality in Catholic moral tradition. According to this principle "all the parts of the human body, as parts, are meant to exist and function for the good of the whole body, and are thus naturally subordinated to the good of the whole body."[186] The roots of this principle are traced to the thoughts of Aristotle and St. Thomas Aquinas.[187] However, the Church has always taught this principle

---

184 Ibid, II, B/5.
185 Brian V. Johnstone, "The Instruction '*Donum Vitae*' and Its Reception," in *Studia Moralia* 26.2 (1988): 223. It seems misleading for Johnstone to refer to the conjugal act in terms of being physically structured. It would be in line with the Church's tradition to say that the conjugal act is the physical expression of the marital intimacy of the couple. This would include the spiritual and the physical dimensions of that sacred and personal act of the married couple. Furthermore, on another point, it is likely and should be understood that the Instruction's use of the terms "goods of marriage" and "conjugal meanings" or "meanings of marriage," all are connected to the *nature* of marriage and should be understood to mean the different aspects of the values and unity of marriage and of the conjugal act. These concepts reveal a historical development of the concepts occasioned by new insights into the nature of marriage.
186 Thomas T. O'Donnell, *Morals in Medicine*, 2nd and Revised Edition (Westminster, Maryland: The Newman Press, 1959), 76.
187 These authors seem to apply this principle differently in limited contexts than it seems to be overstretched today. The principle was relevant for them in the discourse on politics and life in the society. Subsequent literature after Aristotle developed the principle and extended it to justify the mutilation of the body. The Magisterium of the Catholic Church over the years has also made use of this principle. For example, Pius XII in his discourse on "Removal of a Healthy

as pertaining to the physical aspect of man, particularly some specific organs of the body and not in the moral sense as implied in the views of some theologians who tend to over stretch the application of this principle. For instance, in the light of this principle, McCormick like other theologians who argue in defense of the simple case IVF, bases his conviction on the assumption that the significance of the marital act is not limited to any particular sexual act but to the totality of the marital life. He thinks that it is morally incorrect to limit the conjugal act to one particular act, that is, the sexual act. He applies this principle in the moral sense with regards to the conjugal act. McCormick's conviction is that for a child to be the fruit of his parent's love, it must not foreclose the possibility of IVF and ET because for the technique to achieve procreation outside the sexual act is an expression of marital love and indeed an extension of the conjugal act. He agrees with *Donum Vitae* that the child must be the fruit of his parents love but that the sexual act is not the only expression of marital love. In his reasoning, "being a product of a medical intervention is not opposed to being 'the fruit of his parent's love.' "[188] He believes that going extra length to seek a child by means of *in vitro,* a decision taken together between the spouses, is indeed a concrete manifestation of their conjugal love. His argument would suggest that the simple case IVF-ET is a logical and technical extension of love and not a technical replacement. This is based on the reasoning that the human person and his actions combine to give meaning to what pertains to his nature. Consequently, the act of procreation needs not be limited to the specific conjugal act as an expression of love since it does not exhaust all the dimensions that concern conjugal love. Vacek seems to express a similar view when he observes that:

> There are many kinds of love, most of which normally are present in a marriage. Interpersonal bodily intimacy is one kind. The creative hope for a child is a second kind. Cooperation in important activities [such as would be required to

---

Organ" (8 October 1953), used this principle to explain the harmonious relation between the physical and spiritual dimensions of the person. Cited in Monks of Solesmes (ed.), *The Human Body: Papal Teachings* (Boston: St. Paul Editions, Daughters of St. Paul, 1960), 277–279 and in Kevin D. O'Rourke & Philip J. Boyle (eds.), *Medical Ethics: Sources of Catholic Teachings*, 4th Edition (Washington, D.C.: Georgetown University Press, 2011) 306–307.

188 McCormick, *Critical Calling*, 349.

go through homologous artificial reproduction] is a third. An agapic affirmation of a spouse infertility [such as would be required in heterologous reproduction] is a fourth. In addition, there is a myriad of other enactments of love within a marriage. Artificial reproduction does not 'replace' any of these loves, nor need it replace loving sexual acts open to procreation.[189]

Vacek's views as stated are critical of and in response to Berquist who defends the position of *Donum Vitae*'s claim. For Berquist,

> Technology assumes the dominant role when it ... treat[s] the human person as if he existed to be used as a means to the ends proposed by technology rather than exclusively for the expression and fulfillment of his own nature. ... Significant among these properly human activities which are not to be displaced by technology is the act of love in marriage.[190]

Undoubtedly, Vacek acknowledges the validity and strength of Berquist's argument on the special nature of marital love, but he still doubts if marital love is limited in scope to specifically the sexual activity. In the same vein, McCormick considers that the Church's claim that the child is conceived as the product of an intervention of medical or biological techniques and cannot be the fruit of his parent's love as being illogical: *non sequitur*.[191] He expresses the view that the sexual intercourse of the couple is not the only loving act in marriage; this claim is in agreement with Vacek's own position as well.

The argument in support of the simple case IVF and homologous artificial conception in general, emanating from the point of view of the principle of totality seems to hang heavily on marital love. For instance, studying the work of Johnstone in which he details the theological views from other Christian bodies on the reception of the Vatican Instruction *Donum Vitae*, one realizes that they (other Christian bodies) all seem to accept the simple

---

189 Vacek, "Vatican Instruction," 115–116; Marjorie Reiley Maguire, "The Vatican Has Gone Too Far," in *Conscience* 8, 3 (1987), 14–15; Jeanne et Olivier Macherel and Bénédicté et Vincent Fauvel, "Stérilité pour la vie," in *Etudes* 366 (1987): 621–625. Vacek advances his views with the support of the cited works. These authors are in agreement with Vacek against the Magisterium.
190 Richard Berquist, "The Dignity of Human Life and Procreation," in *Crisis* 5, 5 (May 1987): 24–28, at 25.
191 McCormick, "The Vatican Document," 248.

case IVF based on the principle of totality of the marital relationship. The author discerns four basic points that stand in disagreement with the magisterial conclusion on artificial procreation in relation to the simple case, namely:

1. The parental love involved in the search for a child may also be embodied in reproductive procedures.
2. Love-union and procreation must be linked but not necessarily in individual sexual acts but in the marital relationship in totality.
3. Certain technical interventions in procreation maybe considered an assistance/extension of sexual intimacy.
4. Many human activities are imperfect and deprived of their proper perfection, but they are not on this account necessarily morally wrong.[192]

Following the same line of argument that the conjugal act permeates all that the couple do inasmuch as these acts relate to their marriage and not to a particular act, Tauer claims that the availability of alternative reproductive technology might relieve the act of intercourse 'from frustrating preoccupation with vain attempts at procreation and allow it once again to unite the marriage partners in love.'[193] She tends to reason that whatever couples do together as married people cannot be disconnected from the marital life, more so that it pertains to procreation which is essentially one of the goods of marriage. In other words, for Tauer, the marital life incorporates and links together everything the couples engage in insofar as it is by virtue of their marital relationship. The integrity of their marital actions must be evaluated together when talking about the morality of their unity and procreation. She therefore asserts:

---

192 Johnstone, "The Instruction '*Donum Vitae*' and Its Reception," 219. The author rather than supporting these views expressed, he elaborates with great creativity and clarity the seeming errors in these views and a justification of *Donum Vitae*'s conclusions on the simple case. On similar subject of objection to the Catholic magisterial teaching that conception must be the fruit of the specific act of the couple's marital union; See also Kevin T. Kelly, *Life and Love: Towards a Christian Dialogue on Bioethical Questions* (Auckland: Collins Liturgical Publications, 1987).
193 Tauer, "Dissenting Opinions on the Simple Case of In Vitro Fertilization," 139.

> There is no reason why the use of medical techniques to achieve fertilization should contradict the love of the parents. There are thousands of acts of love in marriage, and sex act is only one of them. There is no reason to think that the use of IVF would be an unloving act. It may be the supreme example of the love of husband and wife, as they sacrifice together and work cooperatively in this process with frustrations, hardships, and demands. The joint hardship of treatment for infertility can be an example of enormous self-giving.[194]

Tauer's claim can also suggest that if the couple cannot have a child through the normal means of the conjugal act, that is by the sexual act, they can do so by any other means that is possible and efficient if that is undertaken by virtue of their marital union. She sees no reason why IVF can be classified as an unloving act, when so much sacrifice is involved, a sign of the depth of the spouses' love for themselves and of fulfilling their desire to have a child in their marriage.

Similarly, on this point of argument on the totality of the marital love, that the marital actions of couple towards unity and procreation be held together for a moral judgment on the simple case IVF, one finds a synthesis of this theological opinion in the assertion of Porter. In her opinion,

> A number of moral theologians including, most notably, McCormick, have argued that if we take the new emphasis on the personal and relational (as depicted in *Donum Vitae* and in the works of those who defend its arguments) with full seriousness, it would be difficult to sustain an absolute prohibition on IVF. These theologians readily grant that sexuality has unitive and procreative dimensions that should be held together, but what is critical, in their view is that these dimensions be held together and expressed in the overall relationship between the partners, including its sexual expression over time. For these theologians, it is not necessary to insist that each individual act of sexual intercourse be open to procreation in order to preserve the quality of openness to new life that should characterize the relationship between spouses. Similarly, the act of seeking to conceive a child through IVF can express its parents' mutual, self-giving love, when that act is seen in the context of overall relationship.[195]

Indeed, Porter like other theologians with a similar contrary opinion from that of the magisterial opinion, proposes instead a so-called integral and

---

194 Ibid.,138. See also Vacek, "Vatican Instruction," 115–116; McCormick, *Critical Calling*, 349.
195 Porter, "Human Need and Natural Law," 103. The emphasis in the quotation is not original to the text.

total view of the marital act to encompass every love act of the couple including seeking a child by means of the simple case IVF-ET in the face of infertility.

1.3. On the Moral Object and the Principle of Inseparability of the Conjugal Act

Theological arguments in support of the simple case IVF-ET that the Vatican's Instruction has proscribed reveal the disagreement on the moral object of the conjugal act as the decisive factor for the morality of this reproductive procedure.[196] According to the Catholic Moral Tradition, as

---

196 We understand from Thomas Aquinas, that central to every moral judgment on any human act is the question of what constitutes the object of the action. In the debate on the moral object, there are three views widely held as the common distinction in the understanding of what the moral object of human action consists, but two of these views (the revisionists and neo-scholastics) do not seem to capture correctly Aquinas' teaching on the object of the human act. The new insight of John Paul II in *Veritatis Splendor* is innovative and represents the third interpretation of Aquinas' understanding of the object of the human act. He indicates that "by the object of a given moral act, then, one cannot mean a process or an event of the merely physical order, to be assessed on the basis of its ability to bring about a given state of affairs in the outside world. Rather, that object is the proximate end of a deliberate decision that determines the act of willing on the part of the acting person. Consequently, as the *Catechism of the Catholic Church* teaches, 'there are certain specific kinds of behaviour that are always wrong to choose, because choosing them involves a disorder of the will, that is, a moral evil.'" *Veritatis Splendor*, n. 78. But, in this discussion we do not want to enter into a rigorous inquiry on this matter for there exist controversies among theologians and moral philosophers on what the object of the human act is. This seems basically the point of controversy in the moral evaluation of the simple case IVF-ET. Advocates of this procedure of generating belong to the two groups that are alleged to have misunderstood Aquinas' position or have erroneously interpreted his teaching on the object of a human act. In view of this difficulty, we shall limit our inquiry to what those theologians who reject the magisterial evaluation and conclusion on this hypothetic reproductive procedure maintain. However, it is worthy of note that the disputes over the object of the human act according to some literature can be identified in two general groups: the first group has the tradition of understanding the object of the human act in a physical sense, taking it to be merely an externally visible state of affairs able to be captured

formulated by St. Thomas Aquinas and in recent time reaffirmed by John Paul II in the Catechism of the Catholic Church as well as in the encyclical *Veritatis Splendor*, there are three elements of moral act which together determine the goodness or wrongness of every human act. These elements sometimes called "sources of morality" are: (1) the object chosen, *finis operis*; (2) the end intended, *finis operantis*; and (3) the circumstances surrounding the act.[197] Following the Catholic moral doctrine, it is the object of the moral act that determines the moral quality or species of the act, whereas, the end and circumstances of that act may have impacts on the act.

---

by the third person observer. This first group is linked to neo-scholastic and manual traditions. In the second group, the object of the human act has come to be seen as preconceived notions about what was fitting or is given in a particular situation. Cf. Christopher Kaczor, *Proportionalism and the Natural Law Tradition* (Washington, D.C.: The Catholic University of America Press, 2002), 91–92. Similar to Kaczor's classification, Salzman observes, "Traditionalists maintain that [the object] can designate an external act such that independently of the agent, the act can be considered evil *ex objecto*. Whereas revisionists assert that the moral nature of the external act cannot be determined detached from the human subject, i.e., the concrete situation of an acting, willing, human being." Salzman, *Deontology and Teleology: An Investigation of the Normative Debate in Roman Catholic Moral Theology* (Leuven: Leuven University Press, 1995), 327. However, in addition to the two camps stated above, the research of Duarte Sousa-Lara reveals the third group of interpretation of Aquinas' object of human action. This third group, unlike the first two groups, understands the object of the act as "a proposal of action conceived by the practical reason, which as such has a constitutive relation of agreement or disagreement with the ends appropriate to the human person. The object conceived in this way is in the moral order by its very nature, meaning that the object of the *human act* is, as such, necessarily a moral object." See Duarte Sousa-Lara, "Aquinas on the Object of the Human Act: A Reading in Light of the Texts and Commentators," in *Josephinum Journal of Theology* 15, 2 (2008): 273. This third group consists of contemporary writers who in some unique way differ from the neo-scholastics in their interpretation of Aquinas object of the act but both are distinct from the proportionalist or revisionist interpretation. The new approach brought by John Paul II in *Veritatis Splendor* bears the torchlight of this third group of authors. See also Sousa-Lara, *A especificação moral dos actos humanos seguendo são Tomás de Aquino* (Doctoral Dissertation, Edizioni Università Santa Croce, Rome 2008); Thomas Aquinas, *ST I-II, q. 18, aa. 8–9*; John Paul II, *Veritatis Splendor*, nn. 71–83.

197 Cf. *Catechism of the Catholic Church*, n. 1750; *Veritatis Splendor*, n. 74.

While the object of the act being the nature or species of that act, says a lot about the moral status of that particular act. In line with this doctrine, the Magisterium speaks of intrinsically evil acts, as those human actions which by their objects cannot be rendered good even when their circumstances or/and ends are morally good. It is basically against this type of moral doctrine that the dissenting theologians seem to make their claims. These theologians deny the existence of any intrinsically evil acts. They rather distinguish nonmoral or premoral goods and evils whose moral goodness or badness is determined by weighing the consequences of such actions for moral goods. This is a form of proportionalism or consequentialism, which McCormick as a proponent defends vigorously. He claims that:

> Common to all so-called proportionalists ... is the insistence that causing certain disvalues in our conduct does not by that very fact make an action morally wrong, as certain traditional formulations supposed. The actions become morally wrong when, all things considered, there is not a proportionate reason in the act justifying the disvalue. Thus, just as not every killing is murder, not every falsehood is a lie, so not every artificial intervention preventing or promoting conception in marriage is necessarily an unchaste act.[198]

McCormick like other advocates of the simple case IVF, following the denial of the existence of intrinsically wrong acts, argue that the procedure of the simple case IVF cannot be morally illicit inasmuch as it offers the infertile couple the means to have a genetic child of their own which outweighs the-not-having of a child at all. In other words, human in vitro fertilization is not an intrinsically wrong act as claimed by the Instruction. It is the claim of this theological opinion that the good of having a child is greater and surpasses whatever premoral evil of separating procreation from sexual intercourse. In furtherance of this argument, the dissenting theologians insist that the object of the simple case IVF is what the couple in a particular marriage are set out to achieve, namely to have a child. Generating a child is the object of their act considered together and not simply particular acts considered separately in the whole process. They indicate that inasmuch

---

198 McCormick, *The Tablet* (30 November 1993). Cited in Janet E. Smith, "The Error of Proportionalism," in Edward J. Furton and Veronica M. Dort (eds.), *Ethical Principles in Catholic Health Care* Vol. 1 (Boston, Massachusetts: The National Catholic Bioethics Centre, 1999), 67.

as having a child is a good worth doing and morally obligating of married couple, their action of generating a child with their gametes by means of the simple case IVF cannot be morally illicit.

It can be recalled that John Paul II, expressing the contemporary understanding of the object of a moral action reaffirms in *Veritatis Splendor* that some human actions are morally wrong by their species irrespective of the circumstances and intention of the agent performing the act. The proscription of some techniques of assisted procreation like the simple case IVF is based on this reason. This suggests that the good intended end and the circumstances of infertility involved, do not guarantee the moral goodness of such an act;[199] the act of reproducing human life outside the conjugal act. On the contrary, the dissenting theologians hold that it is erroneous to consider some human actions intrinsically evil without taking note of the circumstances and intention of the infertile couple having the good and noble desire of becoming parents. It is on this ground that these theologians feel that since the good intention of the couple to become genetic parents and the medical agent to serve the need of the couple, as the circumstances of fertility demand it, there is nothing morally wrong in pursuing such a project. This corresponds fittingly to what McCormick indicates: "The physical reality of killing (death= consequence) can be, as inter-subject reality, murder, waging war, self-defense, the death penalty, or resisting insurrection, depending on the circumstances, especially depending on the reason (*ratio*) for which the act is done."[200] McCormick's emphasis on the intention as the goal of the human action explains the reason why he, like others whose views favor proportionalism, insists that the simple case

---

199 John Paul II, *Veritatis Splendor*, nn. 79–83. The document states, "if acts are intrinsically evil, a good intention or particular circumstances can diminish their evil, but they cannot remove it. They remain "irremediably" evil acts; *per se* and in themselves they are not capable of being ordered to God and to the good of the person. 'As for acts which are themselves sins (*cum iam opera ipsa peccata sunt*), Saint Augustine writes, like theft, fornication, blasphemy, who would dare affirm that, by doing them for good motives (*causis bonis*), they would no longer be sins, or, what is even more absurd, that they would be sins that are justified?'" Ibid., 81.
200 McCormick, *Notes on Moral Theology, 1981 through 1984* (Washington, D.C.: University Press of America, 1985), 118.

IVF should not be given a negative moral evaluation. For the dissenting theologians, the factors of infertility (circumstances) of the couple and the good of the child as a blessing of marriage (intention, end) need a particular attention to justify the use of in vitro fertilization in the context of marital relationship inasmuch as care is taken to overcome any avoidable harm in the procedure.

From another perspective, elaborating on the object of the simple case IVF, McCormick proposes two senses that the principle of inseparability of the conjugal act could be read based on the teaching of the Magisterium. According to him, we have both the narrow sense and the broad sense to read the inseparability principle, the principle which defenders of the Instruction use to evaluate the morality of the simple case IVF. The separation of conception from sexual act gives the act of procreation a different meaning. But, McCormick tries to explain that in the narrow sense of understanding the principle of inseparability refers to the connection between the unitive and procreative *in the conjugal act*. That is to say, in the event that if sexual intercourse occurs, these dimensions of unity and procreation entailed in the conjugal act should not be separated. This implies that procreation may be achieved by another means inasmuch as the conjugal act is not affected. Hence, in this sense the artificial procreation is not considered and seemingly not prohibited since the principle is about the protection of the conjugal act.[201] In the broad sense however, McCormick links it with the teaching of Pius XII's discourses on artificial procreation. Here, inseparability of the unitive and procreative aspects of the conjugal act is understood in such a way that fertilization outside the conjugal act is morally wrong and unacceptable. In this sense, in vitro fertilization is excluded.[202] Having proposed the two senses of understanding the

---

201 McCormick, *The Critical Calling*, 337. The author attributes this dimension of understanding the inseparability principle to *Humanae Vitae* of Paul VI and *Familiaris Consortio* of John Paul II.
202 McCormick, *The Critical Calling*, 338. McCormick finds in the two senses of understanding the principle of inseparability of the unitive and procreative dimensions of the conjugal act to development of doctrines. He seems to give the impression that Pius XII's teaching, which is in the broad sense and excludes in vitro fertilization was substituted by the teachings of Paul VI and John Paul II which imply a narrow sense reading of the principle.

inseparability principle, McCormick finds a way to agree with the narrow sense which for him allows in vitro fertilization for the couple inasmuch the gametes are those of the spouses. McCormick's argument in support of the simple case IVF which he occasionally calls standard IVF, partly finds justification based on the above evaluation. Tauer equally sympathizes with McCormick's reasoning as she claims that relying on the principle of inseparability enunciated in *Humanae Vitae* to prohibit contraception, it does not follow in the case of the simple case IVF. Both McCormick and Tauer would have us believe that even if the principle holds true to prohibit contraception, one can approve it without remaining valid in the case of IVF because it is not logically implied.[203]

Furthermore, McCormick equally criticizes the principle of inseparability of the conjugal act as understood and expressed by the Church's Magisterium in *Donum Vitae* and other preceding magisterial documents like *Humanae Vitae* and *Familiaris Consortio*. In his *The Critical Calling*, precisely on the subject of "The Ethics of Reproductive Technologies," McCormick outlines four basic points against the Instruction's understanding of the inseparability of the unitive-procreative dimensions of human sexuality. First, he feels that the idea or notion of every act of sexual intercourse has a procreative dimension as held by the Magisterium can be misleading and cannot be substantiated theologically. He thinks that the document's argument from the principle of inseparability is a weak one to be used to proscribe the simple case IVF. For him, it is not attainable or logically persuasive to attribute a procreative dimension to every sexual intercourse because age factor or the woman's periods are evidence against this position. These are factors that experience and nature have shown to affect fertility and make conception impossible, such that it makes no sense to still maintain that sexual union at those moments be considered "open to procreation" thereby insisting on the inseparability of the unitive

---

203 Cf. Ibid. See also Tauer, "Dissenting Opinions on In vitro Fertilization," 136. Both authors are not concerned with the validity of the argument but its logical sequence in both cases of *Humanae Vitae* and *Donum Vitae*. They both disagree with the Magisterium on its conclusions in both cases of contraception and the simple case IVF-ET.

and procreative dimensions of the conjugal act.[204] And so for him, for the Instruction to insist that there must be in every act of sexual intercourse a procreative dimension implies some form of delimitation and reductionist position. Salzman and Lawler try to support McCormick's claim by indicating that if procreation in a formal sense is extended to include all just and loving acts that always express and give life to the marital union and is not restricted solely to acts of just and loving sexual intercourse that only on occasion give life to a new being, it is not logically clear why procreation in a material sense should not also be extended to include marital acts that are not acts of coitus.[205] For him, the use of this principle to forbid artificial procreation is a misplaced judgment because there is no intrinsic procreative meaning to each and every act of sexual intercourse unless one interprets "procreative" in a metaphorical or formal sense.[206]

Second, McCormick admits that there is some germ of truth in inseparability principle, but that it is a matter of legitimate aesthetic or ecological concern. In other words, it is a matter of integrity of the body different from a moral issue. And so, "all artificial interventions, whether to promote or prevent conception, are a kind of 'second best.'"[207] McCormick feels that

---

204 McCormick, *The Critical Calling*, 348. There is an indication from defenders of the Instruction, which we shall treat in the next chapter on the misinterpretation of the magisterial teaching by McCormick and some other theologians on the principle of inseparability. The claim suggesting that the procreative dimension must be allowed in every act of sexual intercourse is not to be understood in terms of its functionality but in its signification and symbolism. However, the concern of Salzman and Lawler is similar to the document's position than that of McCormick. One thinks that the use of formal and material procreation by these authors makes a distinction between biological (material) procreation and relational (metaphorical or formal) procreation and the concern to understand both positions reasonably legitimate but one that does not seem easy.
205 Salzman and Lawler, *The Sexual Person*, 246.
206 Ibid., 245.
207 Ibid. The Phrase "second best" as used here suggests that either contraception or artificial procreation undertaken within marriage would be an extension of nature and not artificial in terms of anti nature. This implies that such interventions are not contrary to the nature of the marital act but assistance to it. He claims that artificial reproductive technology deprives conception of its perfection but it is better than no conception at all. And of course, imperfection

resorting to integrity as a moral determinant as the Instruction has done gives an impression of a wrong judgment on a moral issue. That is why he refers to it as aesthetic, suggesting that it is not essential in the light of a moral decision. For him, to have a child through an intervention is better than not having at all. Therefore, the prohibition of the simple case IVF-ET is a misplaced judgment.

Third, McCormick questions the rationale behind what he feels is an elevation of an aesthetic-ecological concern into an absolute moral imperative. This point is an extension of the preceding one but with an emphasis on a claim of inadequate biology of the human person on moral norms. He claims the teaching that limits procreation only to the sexual act is adhering to the linear descendant of previous magisterial teachings and rests on inadequate biology that forbids IVF as a means of conception.

Fourth, McCormick indicates that the child being the fruit of his parent's love is certainly adequate as stated by the Instruction. But, what is astonishing and inadequate to comprehend is what he terms "a leap of logic" which makes the sexual intercourse looks like the only loving act in marriage. For him, the child being a product of a medical intervention is not opposed to being the fruit of his parent's love as emphasized by the Catholic Magisterium. He concludes by stating that "I find the congregation's analysis and reasoning on the 'simple case' unpersuasive."[208] His reason for accusing the document's judgment for being unpersuasive lies in the claim that the Instruction's view of the conjugal act is a reductionist view that is inadequate for a balanced anthropological consideration of the person and of his sexuality.

1.4. On the Doctrine of Double Effect and the Conjugal Act

Theologians who argue to defend the simple case IVF directly or indirectly make claims to the principle of double effect. The claim to the principle of double effect in their justification of the simple case IVF is derived from

---

occasioned by the use of technology cannot translate to a morally wrong act simply by the very fact of imperfection as implied in the Instruction.
208 Ibid.

the complexity of the question of artificial procreation.[209] As they apply this principle to the question of procreation outside the conjugal act, they reason that this is the only possible biological means to parenthood for infertile couples. These authors reject the doctrine that identifies certain acts as intrinsically evil or absolutely wrong which we pointed out in the preceding section.

---

209 The Principle of double effect has its historical roots in the medieval natural law tradition, but is particularly emphasized in the thought of Thomas Aquinas. Subsequent Catholic moral theological opinions have affected this principle in its formulation and application. No doubt, there has been a significant controversy about the precise formulation of this principle but in its general sense, it pertains to cases where a particular contemplated or intended action has both good and bad effects. This principle receives its permissibility in the fact that the action is not in itself wrong and does not require that one directly intends the evil result. This principle finds its place in cases of complex moral issues in need of precise decision. Some theological opinions in favor of the simple case IVF seem to directly or indirectly depend to some extent on this principle, when the child is seen as the result that must be achieved at the expense of whatever evil effect (for example, obscuring or blurring the unitive of the conjugal act) involved in the process. Let it be stated that the classical formulation of this principle in Catholic moral tradition requires four basic conditions: first, that the contemplated action must be in itself morally good or morally neutral; second, that the bad result must not be directly intended; third, that the good result not be a direct causal effect of the bad result; and fourth, that the good result be greater or "proportionate to" the bad result. The resort to the doctrine of double effect to support the simple case IVF by some theologians shows the controversy that exists on the true application of this doctrine. For more details see John Paul II, *Veritatis Splendor*, nn. 71–83; Edward J. Furton (ed. et al.), *Catholic Health Care Ethics: A Manual for Practitioners*, 2nd Edition (Philadelphia: The National Catholic Bioethics Center, 2009), 23–26; Peter J. Cataldo, "The Principle of the Double Effect," in *Ethics and Medics* 20 (1995): 1–3; Kevin D. O'Rourke and Philip J. Boyle, *Medical Ethics: Sources of Catholic Teachings*, 4th Edition (Washington, D.C.: Georgetown University Press, 2011), 13–13; Lucius Iwejuru Ugorji, *The Principle of Double Effect: A Critical Appraisal of Its Traditional Understanding and Its Modern Application* (Frankfurt am Main: Verlag Peter Lang GmbH, 1985); Brian D. Scarnecchia, *Bioethics, Law, and Human Life Issues: A Catholic Perspective on Marriage, Family, Conception, Abortion, Reproductive Technology, and Death and Dying* (Toronto: The Scarecrow Press, 2010), 73–83.

The work of Peter Knauer on the theory of double effect gives authors like Eileen P. Flynn some insights for the justification of in vitro fertilization especially in the simple case IVF.[210] Knauer's seminal article was not specifically on artificial procreation but could be considered the cornerstone, the foundation for the school of thought that argues in support of artificial procreation. Knauer had written that "every human act brings evil effects with it. The choice of a value always means concretely that there is denial of another value which must be given as a price in exchange."[211] This interpretation of the theory of double effect informs us of the reason why Knauer's thoughts as well as those who are persuaded by them, argue in defense of the simple case using this theory. For example, Flynn took advantage of Knauer's insights on this theory to argue in support of IVF, indicating that the integrity of the conjugal act can be compromised in order to achieve conception, which is a greater good comparable to the value of the conjugal act. Flyn's understanding of the theory of double effect influenced by Knauer's thoughts, suggests that traditional classification of entire classes of actions, such as masturbation and artificial contraception, as intrinsically evil is not rationally defensible.[212] She agrees with Knauer's view that "one may permit the evil effect of this act only if this is not intended in itself but is indirect and justified by a commensurate reason."[213] In other words, the procreative procedure in the simple case bypasses the conjugal act as lesser evil to achieve the greater good of a child.

Unlike Knauer, Flynn's work on human in vitro fertilization, argues in defense of IVF at least in the case between married couples using the principle of double effect developed by Knauer. She expresses her agreement with Knauer when she writes that:

---

210 Cf. Peter Knauer, "The Hermeneutic Function of the Principle of Double Effect," in Curran-McCormick (ed.), *Readings in Moral Theology, No.1* (New York: Paulist Press, 1979), 2; Eileen P. Flynn, *Human Fertilization In Vitro: A Catholic Moral Perspective* (Washington, D.C.: University Press of America, 1984), 101–118.
211 Knauer, "The Hermeneutic Function of the Principle of Double Effect," 16.
212 Cf. Flynn, *Human Fertilization In Vitro*, 106.
213 Ibid., 20; Knauer, "The Hermeneutic Function of the Principle of Double Effect," 5. Cited in ibid.

> After fifteen years of methodological analysis it would seem that Knauer's assertion of the utility of the principle of double effect and also its corollary that actions described in physical terms not be absolutely prohibited is valid. My acceptance is based on the convincing case Knauer makes regarding the necessity of coming to a decision in moral cases which contain conflicting values, and on my reasoning that God alone is the absolute good, and no human good, such as the sexual act or faculty should be elevated to the level of absolute preference. I realize that in accepting Knauer's thesis I have departed from the first condition traditionally required for the use of the double effect, namely, that the act we intend to perform be good or at least indifferent in its nature; I follow contemporary revisionist moral theology in pointing out that the act need not be good or indifferent, simply because it is a premoral act.[214]

As indicated in the cited text, Flynn rejects the interpretation of the Magisterium that places priority on the object or species or nature of the act of IVF in the determination of its morality. Furthermore, Flynn sustains with some conditions that a decision to become parents of a child through the procedure of human fertilization *in vitro* would have to be made by persons who could reason that there is truly a proportionate reason to allow the ontic evils which are inherent to the technique. These spouses would also have to conclude that the values of marital intimacy and human parenthood would not be weakened should the technique be used as a means of bypassing occluded Fallopian tubes.[215] In employing the theory of double effect to justify procreation by means of the simple case IVF, Flynn's argument corresponds to that of other theologians who feel that the ontic evils inherent in IVF procedure could be permitted or tolerated for the proportionate result of offering married spouses the gift of biological parenthood through their child.

1.5. Summary

In this section we examined some arguments centered on the conjugal act from the perspectives of moral theologians who disagree with the conclusion of *Donum Vitae* on the simple case IVF, and by so doing pointed out their views for the acceptability of this procedure. First, they make claims to the principle of totality, insisting that the conjugal act as a sexual act

---

214 Ibid., 102–103.
215 Ibid., 104.

embraces the entire marriage life of the couples. They claim that it would be a reductionist view to limit procreation to the sexual act even in the case of infertility. In the light of the principle of totality which the dissenting theological opinion claims to apply in procreation, it indicates that bypassing the particular sexual intercourse in order to achieve procreation by means of IVF is in agreement with the Catholic moral tradition which upholds the excision of a particular organ of the body for the wellbeing of the whole body. Since the conjugal act is only an aspect of the marital relationship, it could be morally right to circumvent it if necessary for the good of the spouses to have their genetic child, which can bring fulfillment to their marital union, the wellbeing of the marriage. Secondly, there is the argument on the object of the conjugal act and the claim on the principle of inseparability. Here, they disagree with the traditional determination of the morality of the human act from the object of the act, denying the existence of intrinsically wrong acts.

The Catholic moral tradition teaches that the morality of an action is derived from the object of the act for it specifies the act of the will. This indicates that some human acts are intrinsically evil by their nature or species. Human in vitro fertilization is considered to be one of such human actions. In contrast, following judgment of the dissenting opinion, the simple case IVF can be morally licit bringing together all the factors that warrant its performance, the factor of infertility and the good desire for parenthood. Thirdly, the argument from the principle of double effect was examined. The theological opinion in support of the simple case IVF considers that the particular sexual act which is undermined out of necessity to achieve procreation by means of in vitro fertilization by the married couples would only be a lesser evil in the process of achieving a greater good of a child and of parenthood. In other words, the good of a child and biological parenthood can be proportionate to the natural evil of bypassing the unitive dimension of the conjugal act. These theologians agree with the Magisterium on the importance of the conjugal act but reason that if nature inhibits procreation through it, it could be bypassed as a necessary evil for the good of the entire marriage. On the whole, the dissenting theological view does not affirm or accord the conjugal act the same reverence that the Magisterium reposes on it.

C. Begotten-not-Made

1.1. An Overview

Without delving into the nuances of the terms, it may be important to render the common meanings of these terms: "assistance" and "substitution" in the sense implied in *Donum Vitae*. This could help to evaluate properly the claim that the simple case IVF-ET destroys or diminishes the significance of "begotten" in procreation that employs this technique. The Vatican's Instruction repudiates the simple case IVF-ET with other similar biomedical techniques of human procreation on the grounds that these techniques replace the conjugal act and *ipso facto* implying in this procedure an attitude or a sense of productivity making the child a product of technology and not begetting.[216] In his address to the Bishops of North and Central America and the Caribbean, John Paul II states:

> The technical means which scientists explore cannot be seen as a substitute for the conjugal act but must serve only to facilitate and to help that act attain its natural purpose (cf. *Instruction*, II, 6). Thus it is important to distinguish artificial fertilization from therapeutic techniques which aim at remedying the deficiencies

---

216 *Donum Vitae*, II, B/5. "Conception in vitro is the result of the technical action which presides over fertilization. Such fertilization is neither in fact achieved nor positively willed as the expression and fruit of a specific act of the conjugal union. In homologous IVF and ET, therefore, even if it is considered in the context of 'de facto' existing sexual relations, the generation of the human person is objectively deprived of its proper perfection: namely, that of being the result and fruit of a conjugal act in which the spouses can become 'cooperators with God for giving life to a new person.'" The work of Oliver O'Donovan titled *Begotten or Made?*, is relevant here. O'Donovan's analysis of the concept "beget" in an insightful manner following the sense in which the fathers of the Council of Nicaea conceived of Jesus as the begotten son of God. Discussing precisely the question of artificial procreation, he indicates that to talk of begetting in human procreation is to understand a fact which he says: "Our offspring are human beings, who share with us one common human nature, one common human experience and one common human destiny. We do not determine what our offspring is, except by ourselves being that very thing which our offspring is to become. Just so, the fathers said, the eternal Son of God who was not made, was of the Father's *being*, not his *will*. But that which we make is *unlike* ourselves." O'Donovan, *Begotten or Made?* (Oxford: Clarendon Press, 1983),1.

of nature. We may say that, while infertile couples do not have right to a child, they do have a right to whatever legitimate therapies may be available to remedy their infertility.[217]

John Paul II's remarks reaffirm the Church's teaching that it is not opposed to technology *per se* but it is opposed to those techniques that work against human dignity and the goods of marriage.[218] Thus, the basic criteria for acceptance or rejection of these reproductive techniques are found in the understanding and distinction between "assistance to" and "substitution for" the conjugal act.[219] While the Church's documents judge the simple case IVF to be a form of replacement to the conjugal act, some theologians maintain the contrary opinion. For these theologians, the simple case IVF like any other medical technology that is considered licit, enhances man where nature fails and so can be morally good. The Instruction indicates that when the child is conceived outside the marital sexual act as the product of an intervention of medical or biological technique, he cannot be the fruit of his parent's love. On the section of *Donum Vitae* which evaluates the simple case, the Instruction indicates that homologous IVF and ET is brought about outside the bodies of the couple through actions of third parties whose competence and technical activity determine the success of the procedure. Such fertilization entrusts the life of the embryo to the power of

---

217 John Paul II, "An Address to the Bishops from the North and Central America and the Caribbean on the 7th Bishops' Conference" in Dallas, Texas (25 January 1988), in Donald G. McCarthy (ed.), *Reproductive Technologies, Marriage and the Church* (Braintree: The Pope John Centre, 1988), xv.
218 It is indicated that the principle for the distinction between "assisting" and "replacing" the marital act which *Donum Vitae* makes reference to was first brought into limelight in the Church's Magisterium by Pius XII. This discussion by the Pope inaugurated the way for the possibility of obtaining a biomedical technique worthy of acceptance based on moral requirements. The Pope indicated then that: "although one cannot *a priori* exclude new methods because they are new, yet, as far as artificial insemination is concerned, not only does it call for an extreme reserve, but it is absolutely to be rejected. To say this is not necessarily to proscribe the use of certain means designed only to facilitate the natural act or to assist that act, done in the normal way, to achieve its end." Cf. Pius XII, *Fourth International Congress of Catholic Doctors*, 1954. Cited in *Donum Vitae* II, B/6.
219 *Donum Vitae*, II, B/7.

doctors and biologists, and establishes the domination of technology over the origin and destiny of the human person. The power of the doctors here can refer to the decision and competence required to select or preside over the quality of the embryo to be developed or even for onward transfer to the woman's body. Most significantly, the document concludes that: "such a relationship of domination is in itself contrary to the dignity and equality that must be common to parents and children."[220]

1.2. The Simple Case IVF-ET as Life Enhancing

The Vatican Instruction *Donum Vitae* cautions against treating the child as a product because of the sense of domination inherent and implied in the procedure of IVF and similar techniques of artificial fertilization. The Instruction assumes that all forms of IVF-ET carry with them a meaning that suggests domination and disregard for the dignity of the child. As a critique to this claim, McCormick with other dissenting theologians would insist that such interventions are no more invasive than many other life-saving medical interventions that are considered morally good. They therefore deny that those who seek a child by IVF-ET see the child as a product. Regarding this, McCormick for example, indicates that it is *non sequitur* to accuse IVF of domination, for both prospective parents and medical technologists would not recognize it as such, they would not see it as domination.

A renowned ethicist outside the Catholic circle whose thoughts and works on IVF seem to have influenced greatly some Catholic theologians is Peter Singer. As a strong supporter of IVF, he apparently makes a case for critics of the simple case IVF-ET in one of his articles. He claims that if critics feel that this procedure is "unnatural," then we might be rejecting every modern medicine for the same reason. In his articulation, he regards the simple case to be in accordance with human nature. He observes: "if anything is in accordance with the nature of our species, it is the application of our intelligence to overcome adverse situations in which we find ourselves. The application of IVF to infertile couples is a classical example of this application of human

---

220 Ibid., II, B/5.

intelligence."²²¹ For Singer, when nature seems to work against human nourishing, human intelligence demands that there is need for resistance through the use of medical technology and he describes the simple case procedure as one of such uses of human intelligence. This line of reasoning is synonymous with the theological opinion of some Catholic dissenting theologians on the simple case IVF procedure.

1.3. The Simple Case IVF-ET Technology Accords with Human Dignity

In defense of the simple case IVF-ET, McCormick accuses the Catholic Magisterium of overlooking the whole picture of what artificial procreation is. He believes that there is nothing inhuman about artificial procreation that makes use of the gametes of the spouses, alluding that the technology is equally a product of man, an indeed, an extension of man. McCormick like other defenders of this technique feel that the Creator has endowed man with the ability to master not only the external nature but also his own human nature, as it is evident in many other medical treatments and technologies. And so he sustains that couple who resort to in vitro fertilization and artificial insemination do not see it as manufacture of a product. This is because fertilization happens when sperm and egg are brought together in a petri dish. The technician's 'intervention is a condition for its happening: it is not a cause. For him, "the attitudes of the parents and technicians can be every bit as reverential and respectful as they would be in the face of human life naturally conceived."²²² For him, technology is not anti-human and so its use for procreation should not be condemned or considered morally illicit.

We could make reference here to the observation made by Berquist. He argued that when fertilization is artificially separated from its human

---

221 Peter Singer, "IVF: The Simple Case," in William B. Weil and Martin Benjamin (eds.), *Ethical Issues at the Outside of Life* (Chicago, IL: Year Book Medical Publication, 1987), 44–49 at 45. We have made reference to Singer, a non-Catholic ethicist because of the influence his thoughts seem to have on some Catholic theologians on this matter and particularly for his views that we consider relevant in this work.
222 Ibid.

context, it is reduced to a subhuman level, it occurs in a way suitable for beings without dignity, thereby asserting the domination of technology over the origin of the human person.[223] But in response to his observation, an ally of McCormick, Vacek, avers that medicine is a human activity, and therefore medical fertilization is not "subhuman." He equally observes that, Berquist cannot demonstrate that conceiving a child by genital union or conjugal act is the only way by which humans can be conceived. He would state that the normal way of eating should be done in the human context of feeding through the mouth, but this does not mean that being fed intravenously is a subhuman act.[224]

Similarly, Cahill upholding the position above, argues that acting according to reason by using technologies by couples to achieve what the human nature cannot achieve except by the use of another means is in accord to right reason and therefore morally right. Homologous artificial fertilization of any kind is in accord with human dignity, it is acting in accordance to the natural law because it is reasonable to use it for procreation when couples face infertility challenges. She thinks that morally speaking, there is no essential difference between sexual intercourse and homologous in vitro fertilization. She considers this as beneficial because the couples can realize their shared goal by having a child who is genetically their own provided the technology is used primarily in love and not out of selfishness. She would then have us believe, that the act of procreation, whether it is by in vitro fertilization or by sexual intercourse is moral and in accord with natural law as long as it does not disrupt the couple's marital relationship and does not undermine the couple's shared relation to their children and to the larger society. In the light of this, she sees reproductive technologies as instruments of love and benevolence[225] that are not contrary to dignity of man and the sanctity of matrimony.

---

223 Berquist, "The Dignity of Human Life and Procreation," 24–28, at 25.
224 Vacek, "Vatican Instruction," 116.
225 Ibid., 141–147.

1.4. The Simple Case as an Imperfect Act Not an Immoral Act

To a large extent, the strongest argument in support of the simple case IVF seems to come from the criticism of the principle of inseparability of the two meanings of the conjugal act. Some moral theologians do not believe that for the simple reason that the simple case entails severing the two meanings of the conjugal act, therefore makes it morally wrong and unacceptable. This is in reference to the statement of *Donum Vitae* that "… from the moral point of view, procreation is deprived of its proper perfection when it is not desired as the fruit of the conjugal act, that is to say, of the specific act of the spouses' union."[226] McCormick for instance observes that rendering an action imperfect is not sufficient to make it morally wrong. It is in this light that he believes that generating human life by homologous IVE-ET entails an extension of the conjugal act. He insists that the conjugal love embraces everything the spouses engage in based on their marital union, indeed the whole of their marital experiences. He also notes in a similar context: "Does the separation of the unitive and procreative in an individual act necessarily involve separating the ends or goods of marriage?"[227] For him, the goods of marriage are not hampered or impeded by only a single act that may be necessary for the good of marriage even if it involves the separation of the unitive or the procreative aspects of the conjugal act.

Furthermore, another theologian Tauer, claims to be convinced by the observation of some others who maintain that the availability of alternative reproductive technology might relieve the act of intercourse 'from frustrating preoccupation with vain attempts at procreation and allow it once again to unite the marriage partners in love.'[228] Consequently, the use of medical techniques to assist in procreation that would not have been achieved is not contrary to the couple's love but an extension of it. The acceptance of the sacrifices and burden implied in the procedure is indicative of the strength of the love the couple share and desire to share with the yet to be conceived child.[229] Tauer believes that if the couple cannot have

---

226 *Donum Vitae*, II, B/4.
227 Richard A. McCormick, "Begotten, Not Made," in *Notre Dame Magazine* (Autumn, 1987): 24–25.
228 Tauer, "Dissenting Opinions on In vitro Fertilization," 139.
229 Cf. Ibid., 138. See also Vacek, "Vatican Instruction," 115–116; McCormick, *Critical Calling*, 349.

a child through the normal means of the conjugal act, they can do so by any other procedure that is available provided the choice is made by the couple. From Tauer's line of thought one can presume that she supports the assumption that whatever is technically possible is also ethically right.

Against the Instruction's argument on the subjection of the child to cruelty in IVF, Tauer observes that usually many health issues make one to lose his or her independence before the medical professional or the intervention. And so, she argues that "even with respect to the beginning of life, there are other situations where the medical intervention of medical technology is much more intrusive toward the child than IVF is."[230] She is arguing here that the Instruction's appeal to the intrusive nature of the simple case IVF procedure cannot be a reason against its use because there exist other biomedical devices and services of the same nature in common use but are not morally prohibited. In fact, the dissenting theologians agree that the simple case IVF-ET may not be the ideal or normal procedure for procreation but it does not become morally illicit because of its imperfection. Their argument appeals to the fact that there are many other human activities with deficiency in some sorts but is still not considered morally illicit by the fact of being deficient. Consequently, the argument of the Instruction that the simple case IVF is morally illicit because it deprives human procreation of its perfection is misplaced and disputable.

1.5. Summary

This section articulates the view of several revisionist theologians that the simple case IVF does not portray the child as a product of technology if procreation occurs outside the conjugal sexual intercourse by means of this technique. Against the backdrop of the claim that the child is begotten not made, which judges the simple case in a negative light, some theologians think otherwise. They are of the conviction that the simple case accords with human dignity just as many other medical interventions in human health treatments. For these authors, the simple case does not replace the action of God in procreation as to claim that the child is no longer begotten because the technique is imperfect compared to natural procreation. They

---

230 Tauer, "Dissenting Opinions on In vitro Fertilization," 140.

claim that the action of the medical personnel cannot replace the creative action of God, indeed, man cannot create but God alone.

Secondly, this section has reproduced the arguments of the aforementioned theologians that the artificiality of the simple case technology does not contradict the nature of procreation rather it enhances that which nature lacks in a certain way. And because science and technology are the fruits of human reason and creativity, this technique of procreation merely assists the marital act to realize its goal that is impeded by certain factors of infertility. According to the proponents of this theological opinion, the technique may not be adjudged to be the best, but it is certainly the second best inasmuch as it makes possible the yearning of couples to have children. In other words, the setback of having to use technology to achieve procreation is overcome by the joy of couples becoming parents in the biological sense.

Undoubtedly, what persuades McCormick, Tauer, Cahill, Shannon and others, is the fact that the couple that are in a stable marital relationship, inasmuch as they have agreed to use their gametes to have a child in the simple case IVF procedure, are indeed begetting the child.[231] That is the argument and disposition the dissenting theologians present; they suggest that the stance of the Magisterium that the child is not begotten but made is not convincing enough, in the simple case IVF-ET technology. The dissenting theologians would understand the simple case to meet the requirement of assistance to the conjugal act and not substitution as indicated in the Instruction. The marital relationship in their reasoning is a context by which a child is begotten and this is very much the case in the simple case IVF-ET.

---

231 Indications of this position could be discerned from their expressions. Cf. McCormick, "The Ethics of Reproductive Technology," in *The Critical Calling*, 349: "If experience is our guide – and I think it clearly is not in the congregation's document – accepting medical interventions to overcome sterility between husband and wife is, or can be, precisely a concrete manifestation of their love... I find the congregation's analysis and reasoning on 'the simple case' unpersuasive. So do many others." See also Cahill, "What is the 'Nature' of the Unity of Sex, Love and Procreation?, 147.

Synthesis of the Chapter

In this Chapter Two we explored and presented the theological opinions that consider the simple case IVF-ET as a morally licit means of procreation. In the condemnation of the simple case IVF and other reproductive technologies, the Vatican Instruction makes use of some principles to justify its position. The principle of inseparability of the two meanings of the conjugal act remains the strongest and central principle that *Donum Vitae* uses to justify its proscription of the homologous simple case IVF. In addition, other arguments are also used to complement and strengthen this central principle. Nevertheless, some theologians have criticized the application of this principle in the Instruction and appealed to other principles to justify the simple case IVF as a licit method of procreation. These principles include, the principle of totality, the doctrine of double effect, the supposed proper understanding of the conjugal act, the claim of proper understanding of the natural law theory, the alleged adequate consideration of the human nature.

The dialogue that the Instruction *Donum Vitae* calls for from moral theologians has really been interesting even if it has not always been directed towards accepting the entire teachings of the Magisterium. While some moralists have responded in dissent by way of proposing a contrary opinion on the evaluation of the simple case IVF-ET, many other moral theologians continue to reaffirm the conclusion of the document. The next chapter therefore treats the argument of those who affirm and argue in support of *Donum Vitae* against the simple case IVF-ET.

Chapter Three In Defense of *Donum Vitae*'s Arguments against the Simple Case of Homologous IVF-ET

Introduction

The two fundamental moral questions addressed in the Instruction *Donum Vitae* as presented in Chapter One of this study are evidently indicated in the caption of the document. These questions are: (1) the respect for human life in its origin; and (2) the dignity of human procreation situated within the conjugal act. It is pertinent to recall that in the preceding chapter, we examined some opinions of theologians who have either misunderstood, disagreed or are opposed to the conclusion reached by the Magisterium on the simple case IVF-ET. This is a form of artificial fertilization that is comparatively less complicated or complicit in masturbation and abortive practices, and more so restricted to those in marital relationship. Hence, theoretically, from both clinical and moral perspectives, it appears to be a simple procedure and it is claimed to be free from grave immoral practices unlike the current IVF-ET in practice. From the anthropological and moral dimensions, the Catholic Magisterium on this matter relies on the principle of inseparability of the two meanings of the conjugal act established in man by God to reject this procedure. From this basic principle, the Church teaches that human life is a gift of God to be received, begotten as the fruit of the conjugal act.

Again, according to the spousal significance of the body by which the masculinity and femininity of the man and the woman relate, the child comes as the fruit of that communion between them. It is in the light of these principles and other reasons that some moral theological opinions hail and uphold the conclusion of *Donum Vitae* on the simple case IVF-ET. It is a worthy undertaking to offer some profound theological justification for the moral judgment of the Instruction because the document itself was intended to be a moral guide in the light of new artificial reproductive technologies and not so much a theological treatise. Ratzinger gives a clue to this fact when he notes that the goal of the Instruction is to simply present the responses of Catholic moral doctrine to certain particularly relevant questions regarding new possibilities of intervention, which man has acquired through biomedical technology, in the initial phases of the life of the human being, and the very process of procreation.[232] Therefore, in the following, we will present some of the common arguments and justifications in support of *Donum Vitae* on the simple case in opposition to the claim of dissenting theological opinions within the Catholic circle.

A. The Anthropological Argumentation of *Donum Vitae*

1.1. An Overview of the Argumentation Methodology

In the context of this section, it will be indicated that about human anthropology in relation to sexuality and the generation of human life, the Catholic moral doctrine underscores three questions that require a particular methodology. First, it considers the question of the transmission of human life with particular attention to the principle of inseparability of the unitive and procreative aspects of the conjugal act. The second question concerns the natural continuum that exists in the procreative process. Here, it is a known fact, that procreation is initiated in the conjugal sexual act and if fertile and uninterrupted, conception occurs in the womb and the new life develops gradually for several months, and comes to terms in the birth of the child. As John Sheets description shows, " 'the two-in-one-flesh' nature of the conjugal union describes the whole process as a unified continuum from beginning to its term and its continuation in the nurturing of the child."[233] The Instruction *Donum Vitae* addresses issues that can disrupt this continuum of "two-in-one-flesh unity." Hence, both *Humanae Vitae*

---

232 Joseph Ratzinger, "Preface," in Instruction *Donum Vitae*: *Commentaries and Studies on the Doctrinal Authority of the Instruction Donum Vitae* (Washington, D.C.: USCCB, Libreria Editrice Vaticana, 2013), iii.

233 John R. Sheets, "Christian Anthropology as It Applies to Reproductive and Sexual Morality," in Marilyn Wallace and Thomas W. Hilgers (eds.), *The Gift of Life: The Proceedings of a National Conference on the Vatican Instruction on Reproductive Ethics and Technology* (Omaha: Pope Paul VI Institute Press, 1990), 177; The same article can be found in *Linacre Quarterly* 56, 4 (1989): 23–37.

and *Donum Vitae* employ a similar theological methodology because the questions they address have basic roots: the disruption of new life and the disruption of conjugal union that are naturally designed to be held together in the conjugal act. The third question borders on the intrinsic meaning of the procedure itself apart from other moral issues associated with it.

In fact, the last issue pertains to the dignity of human procreation; one questions if the procedure of IVF respects the dignity of man in his true nature as a being of immense value, spiritual and corporeal in existence. The methodology of the Instruction shows to be faithful to the doctrinal authority of previous magisterial documents and does not claim expertise on scientific and technological matters. This explains why the footnotes and references of the Instruction are evidently in harmony with preceding moral tradition of the Church, authorities and not scientific authorities. Indeed, the document is of a moral and doctrinal nature both in content and approach. While the opposition to the Magisterial would accuse it of appealing to self-authority and not some scientific data, we are called to realize that the Magisterium is simply applying moral principles to issues that pertain to man in his historical and redemptive nature.[234] However, it provides some argumentation to support the principles employed in the text. Joseph Boyle expresses this understanding when he writes that the purpose of the Instruction is not concerned directly with the questions of science and not even with the underlying technological possibilities created by the development of modern biological science. Rather, the interest of the document is on certain human actions that science and technology can influence on the choice of how to generate human life. The use of such scientific and technological knowledge raises serious moral questions. Therefore, it is these moral questions that *Donum Vitae* addresses and not science and

---

234 The biomedical procedures are works of human hands, made for specific applications. The moral teaching of the Church is not on the scientific or technological dimensions of these procedures, in which case the Magisterium would appeal to scientific authorities concerned. But, on the contrary, the Church's concern is on the moral order whereby the choices made in the applications of these technologies for the generation of human life are within the Church's evangelical authority and would be correct to refer to its past and enduring authority where necessary.

technology *per se*.[235] The methodology of the Instruction is of a particular nature on account of the problem it addresses and the authority it operates. Some theologians have tried to formulate more clearly the principles behind the reasoning of the Instruction and one of such earliest scholars to do so after the release of the documents is Boyle. Common experience reveals that the Vatican document requires only a proposal of guidelines on moral issues without establishing the moral principles behind them, the work of deepening the reasoning of such documents belongs properly to theologians. And so Boyle provides five propositions to explain the most basic principles in *Donum Vitae*.

> First, God makes human individuals in His own image and likeness, and He is directly involved in the coming-to-be of each new person. Second, the human person is one being, bodily as well as spiritual, so bodily life and sexuality may not be treated as mere means to more fundamental purposes. Third, every living human individual, from the moment of conception, should be treated with the full respect due a person and so is inviolable. Fourth, sexual activity and procreation can be morally good only if they are part of marital intercourse. Fifth, in marital intercourse, love-making and life-giving should not be separated.[236]

The proposal made by Boyle as stated in the forgoing, succinctly stands to defend the document in its conclusion on the simple case and equally points out the error of the dissenting theologians who consider the simple case as a morally good mode of transmitting human life. The methodology of the document, contrary to the views of the dissenting theologians as seen in the preceding chapter, contains within it indications as developed in the propositions of Boyle. The critique of the dissenting opinion on the methodology of the Vatican document only goes to show the divergence of methodologies on moral issues.

1.2. Argument Based on the Natural Law

The moral criteria for evaluation of medical intervention in human procreation as indicated in the Instruction *Donum Vitae* are based on the anthropological nature of the human person in his unity of body and spirit.

---

235 Joseph Boyle, "An Introduction to the Vatican Instruction on Reproductive Technologies," in *Linacre Quarterly* 55 (1988): 20.
236 Ibid.

The Anthropological Argumentation of *Donum Vitae*   147

These criteria for moral evaluation "are deduced from the dignity of human persons, of their sexuality and their origin."[237] The authors of the document believe that the proper judgment about the medical procedures of human procreation must take into consideration the nature of the person, meaning and purpose of marriage and of sexuality without undermining the origin of human life. These realities have anthropological and moral relevance about anything that concerns the human person. Contrary to the claim by critics of the Instruction that the moral norms of the document were derived from only the biological or physical aspects of the person and based purely on the sex act, one can notice a prior disclaimer explicitly stated in the document itself. From the introductory section of the document, a question about the moral criteria to be used in the field of biomedicine is posed. In response, the anthropological consideration for the unity of the person in his bodily and spiritual dimensions is acknowledged. In so doing, the natural moral law that is exclusive to rational creatures is being considered the appropriate law guiding human actions because by nature man is created to participate in the eternal law of God by virtue of being the crown of creation and being created in the image and likeness of God. This natural moral law which is the same as natural law:

> Expresses and lays down the purposes, rights and duties which are based upon the bodily and spiritual nature of the human person. Therefore, this law cannot be thought of as simply a set of norms on the biological level; rather it must be defined as the rational order whereby man is called by the Creator to direct and regulate his life and actions and in particular to make use of his own body.[238]

The authors of the document had foreseen the misunderstanding that might be read into the judgment of the document by pre-empting with this clarification but still the document is criticized by some theologians for being biologically based as we have seen in the preceding chapter of this work.

However, many moral theologians faithful and conversant with the Church's moral doctrine have written to defend among other things that the Instruction's natural law application is not physically based but that its natural law is in conformity to the true nature of the person as body-soul

---

237 *Donum Vitae*, II, B/7.
238 *Donum Vitae*, Introd., 3. See also Paul VI, Encyclical Letter *Humanae Vitae*, n. 10.

being. Expatiating on the natural moral law employed in *Donum Vitae*, John M. Haas explains that:

> The morality of an act is not determined in light of its conformity to some physical law of nature but rather of its conformity to or consonance with the reasonable nature of the acting person. The question of artificiality being a moral determinant is not even raised.[239]

He goes on to state that the moral determinants for the document are certain values, meanings and goods 'of personal order,' not the natural order. These goods as the document indicates concern the life of the person called into being and the special means of generating this life that corresponds to the dignity of the person. Equally, commenting on this matter, Sgreccia makes two points of clarification that are worthy of note here: (a) The 'nature' that the Catholic Magisterium mentions in its documents and for which it demands respect is not automatically biological nature (*bios*) alone, but nature in the metaphysical sense: the structural peculiarity of the human person thanks to which the human person is what he is, an individual in whom spirit and body are united in such a way that the spirit manifests itself in the body and the spirit informs, structures, and vivifies corporality. Hence, nature is what constitutes the human person in his uni-total essence. (b) The law that the Catholic Magisterium mentions in the documents is the natural *moral law*, not a physical and biological law. The biological law is always obeyed, even in artificial procreation, because if it were not observed in combining the male and female gametes, there would be no fertilization; what is not being observed is the natural *moral law*, which obliges us to consider man as a person in his totality and the procreative sexual act as the expression of the spirit and of personal love in the giving of one's corporality. Therefore, "what is being condemned is not technology *per se*, nor the application of technology to the human body, but rather the fact that this type of application introduces a dualism by separating the biological-fecundatory dimension from the spiritual dimension of the spousal 'self.'"[240] Obviously, Sgreccia's commentary and insightful inputs on the understanding of the natural law which the Instruction refers to,

---

239 Haas, "The Natural and the Human in Procreation," 105.
240 Sgreccia, *Personalist Bioethics*. 486–487.

seem to respond to the critics who have alleged that the Instruction's derivation of moral norms constitutes an error on its judgment about certain reproductive techniques especially the simple case of homologous IVF-ET.

In fact, in defense of the Magisterium, some theologians also claim to have a better picture and understanding of the Church's teaching on the rejection of the simple case IVF-ET and they have tried to show this with inspiration from the Magisterium. The Instruction reveals itself to be in line with the tradition of the Magisterium's teaching on marriage. Like the teaching of Pius XI on Marriage, *Casti Connubii*, which points out certain errors of some people on the intrinsic structure of marriage, it emphasizes that marriage has a meaning and purpose established by God and guided by some laws. And so whatever is in accordance with the nature of man and promotes his wellbeing in this plan is good, but that which is against that nature and degrades it is intrinsically evil. This is precisely the same conclusion of *Donum Vitae*. According to John Gallaher, in the context of the Church's teaching, "being according to nature" is to be determined not by considering the physical aspect by itself but by looking at the nature and purposes of marriage.[241] In the light of the teaching of John Paul II, the human body is the medium by which the human person acts. In his series of Wednesday audience catechetical discussions on human love and sexuality now called "The Theology of the Body," John Paul II teaches us the truth of the person by emphasizing that the body is not simply a "container" of the person but an intrinsic dimension of his being without which he cannot be said to exist in the world. In other words, the human body is the person: that is his being, nature and form. This is radically opposed to the Cartesian dualism where only the "thinking self" or consciousness is said to identity the person. Perhaps, this account for the reason why it is easy to erroneously accuse the Magisterium of being physicalistic in its derivation of moral norms on sexual morality because of its consideration for the body.

Furthermore, the defending theological view has insisted that the argumentation of the Instruction makes human biology morally relevant in a

---

[241] John Gallagher, "Magisterial Teaching from 1918 to the Present," in *Human Sexuality and Personhood* (St. Louis: Pope John Center, 1981), 196.

way that is adequate. The adequacy is based on the idea that human biology is about the person. For example, Johnstone writes,

> In the teaching of the Instruction, human biology is morally relevant because it is of the person. It will be remembered that the first major step in the argument is to link the meanings of the human realities of sexuality and marriage with the divine. The second major step is to link these meanings to bodily structures and physical acts. Here the link is provided by the philosophical, anthropological thesis of the union of spirit and body.[242]

Johnstone submits here that intervention on the human body cannot be without touching the person in some essential way, because the person cannot be without the physical body. However, he notes that the union of soul and body does not make explicit for us to know the particular structures of the human body that are morally relevant, nor how they are morally relevant. In view of this, there would be another supporting thesis. In the reasoning of Johnstone, the second argument that is capable of defending the preceding one is expressed thus:

> The goods of marriage (love-union and procreation) as goods of the spirit, are, at the same time, embodied values, that is, values realized in and through the physical structures of the human body. The particular physical structure in which these goods are realized is the conjugal act. The 'meanings' of the act derive, then, from the goods that act is designed to realize, that is love union and procreation.[243]

The structure of this argument could be summarized in another way following the suggestions of Tettamanzi. For him, this argument is a multilevel structure, where levels are linked to other levels as symbols of expressions. Here, the element of symbol is brought to play a significant role in the understanding of this complex structure. At the highest level is the giving love of God. This is symbolized and expressed in the giving and reception of love of the couple, which is a participation in the divine love. That is,

---

242 Johnstone, "The Instruction *Donum Vitae* and its Reception," in *Studia Moralia* 26, 2 (1988): 222. The author makes reference in his footnote to Dionigi Tettamanzi, "Fecondazione artificiale e 'immagine di famiglia,'" in Elio Sgreccia (ed.), *Il dono della vita: istruzione della Congregazione per la dottrina della fede su il rispetto della vita umana nascente e la dignità della procreazione umana* (Milan: Vita e Pensiero, 1987), 141.
243 Johnstone, "The Instruction *Donum Vitae* and its Reception," 223.

The Anthropological Argumentation of *Donum Vitae*

This giving is symbolized and expressed in the logic of the body, which in turn is expressed and concretely in the act of the sexual intercourse. The normativity of each level of structure derives ultimately from the normativity of divine love itself. It could thus be argued that homologous artificial fecundation violates the normative human structures which are normative as participations in the divine.[244]

From here, we can see that the argumentation is not solely dependent on the physical aspect as claimed by some theologians. In fact, no one doubts the biological dimension of the person in respect to the sexual act. This goes to illustrate that the emphasis on the biological aspect of procreation is in respect of the structure of the nature of procreation as man's response to the expression of God's love to man. It is not easy to interpret and formulate moral norms on the question of human sexuality without emphasizing anthropologically the norms of procreation deriving from natural law as done in *Donum Vitae*. The Instruction in the light of the basic principle of inseparability first explicated by Paul VI, recognizes "the laws inscribed in the very being of man and woman."[245] In the thinking of Johnstone, the laws referred to in the citation can be the biological laws and these laws are not contrary to moral norms of procreation. It is because of the physical, biological structure that the conjugal act has the potentiality of transmitting a new human life. In other words, the generation of life is dependent upon the biological laws inherent in man and woman, such that given a favorable condition, the union of the gametes of the man and woman in sexual intercourse can naturally lead to fertilization. This point is emphasizing the biological laws and not moral laws. However, Johnstone wants to indicate that the biological laws are still relevant in the derivation of moral laws that guide human procreation.

There is still yet to demonstrate how and why the physical, biological structure of the marital act is morally relevant and why it would be erroneous to interpret the document's derivation of norms for procreation from purely physicalistic category. Johnstone defends the document by

---

244 Tettamanzi, "Fecondazione artificiale," 143: "In tale senso la fecondazione artificiale omologa, violando la logica dell'amore di donazione totale – quindi anche del corpo – degli sposi, viola l'amore a la donazione coniugale *in quanto* participazione all'amore donato di Dio in Cristo." (Emphasis is added). Cited in Johnstone, "The Instruction *Donum Vitae* and its Reception," 223–234.
245 *Donum Vitae*, II, B/4, a.

noting that the text of the Instruction specifically rejects arguments from the analogy between human biology and that of lower forms of life. Therefore, biology is not relevant here because it indicates 'what nature has taught all animals' as Ulpian would have it. The argument of the document does not attempt to derive the moral norms governing human procreation from analogies from lower forms of life. Hence,

> The basis of the position is therefore, not a 'biologistic' interpretation of natural law. That is, it is not argued that the biological structure of acts is relevant because that is the normal pattern, where normal means usual for 'all animals.' Rather, the Instruction refers to '… the rational order' by which human agent is to be guided.[246]

It is indicated that the rational order the Instruction refers is synonymous with the natural law and not the law of nature. The laws of nature are descriptive. They describe what happens time after time given the same conditions. These laws govern every created thing without distinction. But, the natural law is prescriptive, it prescribes what ought to be done because it accords with human nature and enhances human life. It is a moral law directing human conducts, human actions according to their purposes. The natural law is applicable only to rational and free beings, to humans alone. The natural law guides and directs man in such a way that he consciously acts according to the ordinance of reason for the common good as designed by God the Creator and Ruler. The understanding of this order of things is underscored in the Instruction when it states, "…the natural moral law expresses and lays down the purposes, rights and duties which are based on the bodily and spiritual nature of the human person."[247] From this reasoning, it could be deduced why the simple case IVF is judged to be a morally wrong means to generate human life. The choice to generate human life outside the conjugal act defects from God's design and fails to treat procreation as a symbol of God's love for man, the love that is lived by spouses which capacitates and leads them to the generation of life as a fruit of mutual gift of themselves. Besides, the order of realizing this mission of being co-creators with God implied in the natural law and taught

---

246 Johnstone, "The Instruction *Donum Vitae* and its Reception," 224–225. The internal reference is from *Donum Vitae*, Introd., 3.
247 *Donum Vitae*, Introd., 3.

by the Magisterium cannot be realized in the simple case IVF-ET because fertilization is not the fruit of the specific act of conjugal sexual union but as the result of technical expertise of medical personnel.

1.3. The Unity of the Human Person Adequately Considered

The moral teaching of the Magisterium as presented in *Donum Vitae* is based on the various aspects of *unity* of the human being. These various aspects of unity are the foundation for any right judgment of any technique of artificial procreation. First, we talk of the unity of the person as a composite being of body and spirit. Second, we consider the unity of the two meanings (love-union and life-giving or procreation) of the conjugal act. Third, we can also look at the unity of actions naturally meant to be a continuum for procreation (from conjugal sexual intercourse = fertilization = development = birth). All of these dimensions flow from the anthropological structure of the human being and of procreation. While the critics of *Donum Vitae* claim that the anthropological consideration in the document is physicalistic and inadequate, the defenders of the Instruction reject this claim and allege instead that the dissenting theologians lack accurate understanding of the document's argument.[248]

Proponents of the document claim that in order to show the true reading of the content and doctrine of the Instruction, it is pertinent to indicate briefly that the critics of the Instruction are in error on three vital points. Firstly, that the critics have inadequate hermeneutics of the principles of the Magisterium. Secondly, that the critics' proposal that procreation be placed within marital relationship as a whole without specifying the relevance

---

[248] Some scholars feel that the rejection of the Instruction's teaching to be inaccurate has its antecedent. "It is a mistake, therefore, to suppose that one can find in the Instruction an attempt to persuade those who reject its principles. Since dissenting theologians and many outside the Church rejects at least some of these principles, it is not surprising that the Instruction has been found unpersuasive by many. But that is no criticism of the Instruction." Cf. Boyle, "An Introduction to the Vatican Instruction on Reproductive Technologies," 22. This suggests, as it is implied in Boyle's observation, many theologians who do not find *Donum Vitae*'s teaching persuasive are those who are systematically opposed to some of the moral principles of the Magisterium beyond the current document.

of the conjugal act, reduces or at most makes procreation an impersonal act. Thirdly, defenders of the anthropology of the Magisterium insist that the emphasis of the dissenting opinion on the spiritual aspects of man is a misconception of the true nature of man and it has implications suggesting that the physical body of the person is morally irrelevant in the derivation of moral norms on sexuality and procreation.

Furthermore, to attenuate the argument of the critics and clarify the teaching of the Magisterium, some theologians show that *Donum Vitae* in accordance with the Church's vision of man explicitly states that any moral evaluation of biomedical technologies must be based on the truth of man in his bodily and spiritual dimensions. In the introductory section of the Instruction, its authors did not forget to recognize the unified totality of man as a distinct being from other creatures. When the Instruction asks for the moral criteria to be applied to the problem of artificial procreation, it indicates that such criteria must correspond to the true nature of man. In the light of this, Donald P. Asci writes,

> *Donum Vitae* puts forward a vision of man in which the substantial union of the human body and soul is significant not only for describing who man is but also for determining how man is 'to direct and regulate his life and actions and in particular to make use of his body.' Thus, the very nature of man serves as a reference point for his moral decision – making. Yet, it is not only his identity that possesses moral significance for man but also his vocation. In addition to the norms of the natural law, God 'has inscribed in man and woman the vocation to share in a special way in His mystery of personal communion and in His work as Creator and Father.'[249]

By the fact of recognizing the true constitution of man as a composite being of body and soul, *Donum Vitae* reveals why the generation of life cannot be equated with other creatures and much more why the procreative process should not be treated as merely a biological affair.

For Sgreccia, the theme of corporeity expressed in *Donum Vitae* is very relevant inasmuch as it says so much about man who is both temporal and transcendent. He explains that by corporeity is understood in the

---

249 Donald P. Asci, *The Conjugal Act as a Personal Act: A Study of the Concept of Conjugal Act in the Light of Christian Anthropology* (San Francisco: Ignatius Press, 2002), 157. The internal quotation is from *Donum Vitae*, Introd., 3.

Instruction as well as in contemporary biological and philosophical sciences as a "manifestation, epiphany, language of the person, particularly with regard to sexuality in the male and female relationship."[250] He goes on to explain that the unity of the human being and the unity of the body and spirit are corroded in the use of artificial means to generate human life. Again, in the discussion of the Christian anthropology as it applies to reproductive and sexual morality, another theologian, Sheets gives an impressive outline to understand the anthropological argumentation in the Instruction contrary to the claim of critics. Making reference to *Humanae Vitae*, he admits that the said document as well as *Donum Vitae*, contain an adequate picture of man in light of its moral judgment. For him, these magisterial documents point out that the moral evaluation of reproductive questions has to be sought within the context of a total vision of human existence. He notes that *Humanae Vitae* indicates that the problem of birth, like every other problem connected to human life is to be considered beyond partial perspectives of either the spiritual or the physical. In the same way, *Donum Vitae* calls for the necessity of keeping in view the unified totality of the human person as it concerns intervention in human procreation. Therefore, it can be said that:

> This method of argumentation might be called the argument of 'intrinsic coherence.' The whole network of relations that constitute the identity of the human person has its intrinsic laws. The violation of one of these laws leads to a disequilibrium that weakens and distorts the coherence of the whole.[251]

This analysis points out why the generation of human life outside the conjugal act or bodily union of the spouses constitutes a moral problem.

From another perspective, Sheets speaks of Christian anthropology, suggesting that the reality of Christian faith brings a new meaning in the life of the human person and this dimension is only found through revelation. In other words, the true nature of the person in the light of his destiny can be known with the help of revelation. Sheets explains:

> Through revelation we know there is more at work in the heart of man, in the world of things, in the events of history than can be discovered by reason.

---

250 Sgreccia, "Moral Theology and Artificial Procreation," 130.
251 Sheets, "Christian Anthropology," 178.

Revelation is precisely that light, picked up by faith, which illumines the whole meaning of man, both his mystery as a graced person as well as his enigmatic character as carrying with him the effects of both personal as well as original sin.[252]

Therefore, the methodology of evaluating the reproductive techniques cannot overlook this dimension of Christian faith, because faith changes the whole meaning, existence and destiny of the human person. Because the human being is created in the image and likeness of God, the Christian Faith sheds light on the nature of man as a transcendent being who cannot be understood adequately by scientific methodology only. Empirical science is lame in that dimension of humanity that speaks of the Divine Being and the destiny of man in relation to Him. It is therefore with faith made possible by revelation that the true assessment of the nature of the human being and of his actions can be achieved. The Vatican Instruction shows laudable evidence of its attention to this reality in the rejection of certain means of intervention in human procreation. It is in line with this that the Instruction points out that parenthood is a vocation to share in the Fatherhood of God the Creator.[253] In fact, without the Christian faith founded on revelation, it will be impossible to grasp the truth of the message expressed in the document. The Instruction appeals to this truth when it refers to the biblical account of human origin; man being created in the image and likeness of God, suggesting that the origin, existence, essence and destiny of man depend on God's plan and the economy of salvation. Therefore, science and technology as inventions of man have their limits with regards to the origin and existence and destiny of the human person as well as the institution of marriage.

Janet Smith's views to support the teaching of the Magisterium on the simple case are also profound. According to her, when *Donum Vitae* asserts that the transmission of human life has a special character of its own, which

---

252 Ibid., 177.
253 *Donum Vitae*, Introd., 1: "The gift of life which God the Creator and Father has entrusted to man calls him to appreciate the inestimable value of what he has been given and to take responsibility for it: this fundamental principle must be placed at the center of one's reflection in order to clarify and solve the moral problems raised by artificial interventions on life as it originates and on the process of procreation."

derives from the special nature of the human person,[254] the special nature of man here indicates his bodily and spiritual dimension which makes him different from lower animals. For her, this principle stated above shows the weakness and limitation of the argument of the dissenting theologians against *Donum Vitae*, which claims that the Church's judgment is physicalistic or biologistic in her view on sex. She thinks that it could rather be said that the Church has a Personalist view of sexuality. Otherwise, it would permit methods and procedures used in horticulture and animal husbandry for the transmission of human life.[255] Smith's submission is an affirmation of the teaching of *Donum Vitae*, that the human body is a personal body and not a sub-personal or impersonal property, the person's identity cannot be known outside his body. This personal dimension that is part of the essential nature of the human person, has a role in the formation of moral norms. The fact that man's bears the image and likeness of God, who creates out of love, in love and for love, makes procreation an act of responsibility whereby each and every human life should be the result of a personal and conscious act of love between man and woman. The anthropological nature of the spouses in their masculinity and femininity bears this truth and it is in recognition of this fact and its theological import that the Church reaffirms in *Donum Vitae* the special nature and dignity of procreation.

1.4. The Human Role in Procreation and the Logic of *Donum Vitae*

The logic of *Donum Vitae* is characteristic of Catholic moral doctrine and this is deeply rooted in Christian anthropology. The central teaching of the document is that human life is a gift from God that has been entrusted to men and women, who are called to appreciate its inestimable value and take responsibility to promote its dignity with regard both to the human being called into existence and to the special nature of the transmission of human life. The Vatican document indicates that the coming into existence

---

254 *Donum Vitae*, Introd., 4. This point is in consonant with the teaching of *Mater et Magistra* which condemns the use of certain methods and means for the generation of human life, means that could be appropriate for transmission of the life of plants and animals. Cf. *Mater et Magistra*, III, 447.
255 Janet E. Smith, "The Vocation of Christian Marriage as an Approach to the Bioethics of Human Reproduction," in *The Gift of Life*, 54.

of human life is not ultimately subject to the will of man but to his cooperation; life belongs to God ultimately. This is the logic of the Instruction that is applied to new methods of intervention in human procreation. This logic is found in the opening paragraph of the Instruction when it hints that man is called to responsibility in the transmission of life: "The gift of life which God the Creator and Father has entrusted to man calls him to appreciate the inestimable value of what he has been given and to take responsibility for it."[256] In this statement, there are three fundamental elements that cannot be overlooked in the evaluation of the morality of the simple case IVF. First, life is a gift from God the Creator and by implication, He is properly the owner of human life, He alone has absolute power over its origin and existence. Second, human life is entrusted to man. This means, it is a gift for custody and man is merely a custodian and has no absolute power over it. And by virtue of being a custodian, man is called to take responsibility for life both in its origin and existence. This responsibility is man's vocation to share in the life of God. In every act of procreation, God re-enacts the act of creation and in this case with the cooperation of man. Third, human life has intrinsic worth, inestimable value or dignity that transcends apparent realities. These basic indications in the Instruction are essential in the methodology employed by the Magisterium in the assessment of artificial interventions in human procreation.

Undoubtedly, the transmission of human life is not purely God's act alone as in the creation of the first man, Adam. Procreation is not an instinctual or contingent act whereby man does not have any control, it is a human act consciously and freely undertaken in response to God's call. It is different from the reproduction that occurs among lower animals where the aspect of responsibility is absent because of the lack of the quality of rationality. In fact, for man, the "creative act of divine donation takes place in the context of human sexuality and is a work of both God and man. In accordance with the personal nature of man and the dignity of the human person, God does not use man's sexuality in a passive manner."[257] The action of the couple

---

256 *Donum Vitae*, Introd., 1.
257 Asci, *The Conjugal Act as a Personal Act*, 175. This citation makes reference to: Gino Concetti, *Sessualità, amore, procreazione* (Milan: Edizione Ares, 1990), 115: "La creazione del primo uomo e della donna è esclusiva opera

in the transmission of human life is not passive and should not be made to appear that way. Procreation requires naturally a co-operation with God to bring about new human life. The argument of the Instruction on human procreation takes serious this fact when it insists that reproductive technologies are not neutral inasmuch as they are products of human hands. Their inventions and uses reveal the intentions of their manufacturers and end users. The Magisterium believes that these procedures *per se* have inherent meanings that contradict the role of the spouses in procreation. They make the spouses' role passive and non-essential, this in turn has inherent implications for both the couple and the child born from such procedures. And indeed, the most central role that does not require to be substituted is the conjugal sexual act and this is conspicuously bypassed in the simple case IVF procedure. As the document clearly states, that human procreation requires on the part of the spouses responsible collaboration with the fruitful love of God; the gift of human life must be actualized in marriage through the specific and exclusive acts of husband and wife, in accordance with the laws inscribed in their persons and in their union.[258] In the light of the above indication, we can see affirmation of the truth that in the natural order there are laws inscribed in the being of man to regulate his actions by virtue of being a rational creature and likewise there are moral principles that regulate marital union in conformity with the nature of the person.

To underscore the importance of the role of the spouses in the generation of life, Smith argues that although God is the true Creator of each

---

di Dio; la generazione dei discendenti è opera dell'uomo e della donna in collaborazione con Dio." See also John Paul II, *Letters to Families*, n. 9: "In affirming that the spouses, as parents, cooperate with God the Creator in conceiving and giving birth to a new human being, we are not speaking merely with reference to the laws of biology. Instead, God alone is the source of that 'image and likeness' which is proper to the human being, as it was received at Creation. Begetting is the continuation of creation." This is an apt description of what the Magisterium teaches by calling man's attention to some procedures of artificial procreation that work contrary to the collaboration that requires in human procreation.

258 *Donum Vitae*, Introd., 5. This citation reflects the teaching of the Vatican Council document, *Gaudium et Spes*, n. 50.

and every human life, the role of the parents is neither unimportant nor simply mechanical.[259] This indicates that according to God's design, man and woman are to participate in the transmission of human life as persons, as "human beings made of flesh and blood, endowed with minds and hearts."[260] This explains that the couple perform an active and significant role in conformity with their nature, dignity, freedom and vocation as married persons. *Donum Vitae* informs that although the couple's role is active and significant in the transmission of life but this does not supplant the primary role of God. The role of the parents is secondary to God's yet essential and in collaboration with God's. Therefore, man is not the master of procreation but simply its "servant" in the service of life.[261] Reflecting on human role as being collaborative with God in the transmission of life, Asci outlines three principal ideas about this fundamental truth. (1) Man and woman alone cannot generate a child; (2) man and woman must be co-subjects with God in the transmission of life, meaning that they must actively do something with God; and (3) as co-operators, the behavior of man and woman is modeled upon and corresponds to that of the principal agent, namely, God.[262] The above lines of thought serve to indicate the theological and anthropological reality in the event of procreation upon which *Donum Vitae*'s judgment is considered by many theologians as adequate and persuasive against other contrary views.

Another area in the Instruction deserving attention as part of its methodology would be that of freedom and responsibility both on the part of the couple and the biomedical technologists. This freedom has foundation in the truth of man's nature. The Catholic Magisterium understands that the generation of human life which God the author of life commits on trust to man, demands human freedom and wisdom to discern the truth of human nature. This gives a clue to the "no" response of the Magisterium to certain procedures of artificial procreation that do not conform to the natural order proper to man. Caffarra hints that there are three postulations concerning the existence of human life, two of which exemplify the ruin

---

259 Smith, "The Vocation of Marriage," in Boyle, *Creative Love*, 126.
260 Pius XII, *Allocution to the Union of Italian Catholic Midwives*, 1949.
261 *Donum Vitae*, II, B/4. c.
262 Asci, *The Conjugal Act as a Personal Act*, 176.

of freedom and could be possible motivation for or against the simple case IVF-ET procedure. The first assumption says that human life is a product of *chance*; another one says each human being is the fruit of an inexplicable *necessity* and the last explanation says every human being is the fruit of a free act of God's *creative love*. For him, to affirm that we have come into being by chance makes it impossible, with any consistency, further, to affirm the presence of an indestructible meaning of our existence. To affirm the necessity of coming into being makes it impossible, with any consistency, to affirm the existence of a reason for which it is worthwhile living, a reason more important than life itself.[263] He goes on to explain that "to affirm a divine creative act at the origin of our coming into being leads to the further affirmation of a dependence on God that is radical [that concerns the very act of being], a dependence into which the human subject is called to enter more profoundly in order not to fall into the nothingness from which it was drawn."[264] Caffarra believes that it is in the space opened up within this threefold explanation that *free will* is called to make a decision and to decide the supreme destiny of the person.

The indication made by Caffarra expresses the logic implied in any form chosen by man to generate life. Procreation being man's cooperation with God's creative love, morally requires that man's freedom in this regard should correspond to the divine law inscribed in man's nature.[265] The creative act of God and the procreative act of the couple can be said to have a significant common point in the act of conjugal sexual intercourse. In the light of this, Caffarra submits that:

> The exercise of conjugal sexuality, when it is fertile, constitutes the mysterious tangential point between the created universe of being *and* God's creative love; it is even the point at which this creative love comes *within* the created universe of being, with a view to the *new* term of its potency.... The fertility inherent in the conjugal act is not a merely biological fact. It brings the spouses, objectively,

---

263 Carlo Caffarra, "Who is Like the Lord, Our God?" in Janet E. Smith (ed.), *Why Humanae Vitae was Right: A Reader* (San Francisco: Ignatius Press, 1993), 256.
264 Ibid.
265 Cf. *Gaudium et Spes*, n. 50.

into a real relationship with God the Creator, whether or not they are conscious of the fact.[266]

All that the forgoing attempts to express is that in human procreation, man and woman who have been married, express their freedom to procreate only within the plan of God who is the author of life.

In the same vein, Livio Melina in his thoughts on this debate recognizes the fact that the spouses, who have the obligation to ask and receive the gift of children from God, do so as collaborators. They acknowledge that it is from God that the initiative to generate human life has significance. A man and a woman, in generating, truly collaborate with God, from whose creative initiative, as the Church believes, takes its immediate origin the spiritual soul of every human person, created in His image and called in Christ to freely take part in God's life, an act that is indeed godly.[267] Similarly, the submission of Ratzinger appeals to Melina when he makes reference to him by saying that "… rather than the mere 'reproduction' of an example of the species, one should speak of the 'procreation' of a unique and unrepeatable person who is called to a special relationship with God."[268] The idea here is that, beyond the bodily dimension of the procreative process, the divine breath is inevitable. It is like saying: in every procreative event the creative breath of the first man is re-enacted. God therefore is always invisibly active in human procreation and so technical procedures must not overturn what is befitting of man in relation to God. In this light,

> It should be made immediately clear that when it is stated that the human marriage partners are collaborators with God in the generation of a new human being the intention is not to limit their role to the mere physical sphere. The generation of

---

[266] Caffarra, "Who is Like the Lord, Our God?," 257. Caffarra was actually addressing the problem of contraception as tackled in *Humanae Vitae*, but since the basic law that deals with contraception is the same with that of artificial procreation it is in place to apply it to both problems.

[267] Livio Melina, "The Intrinsic Logic of Interventions in the Field of Human Artificial Procreation: Ethical Aspects," in Juan De Dios Vial Correa and Elio Sgreccia (eds.), *The Dignity of Human Procreation and Reproductive Technologies: Anthropological and Ethical Aspects* (Vatican City: Libreria Editrice Vaticana, 2005), 114.

[268] Ibid., 115. The author makes reference to Joseph Ratzinger, "Uno sguardo teologico sulla procreazione umana," *Medicina e Morale* 38 (1988), 507–521.

a person, *corpora et anima unus*, is a unitary event in which the spiritual level occurs in simultaneous unity with the corporeal level.[269]

Furthermore, Melina insists that God would not wish that the child be born outside the embrace of a father and a mother. It could obviously happen that biomedical technology manipulates or exploits the natural course of procreation to have a child, but this would be morally illicit. It would be bereft of the proper dignity and reverence that is associated with human procreation. Thus, divine authority does not authorize from outside the paternal and maternal authority of the human parents but becomes the limit that is its foundation from within, and in forming its foundation it governs its exercise. Parenthood has the form of a 'vow,' that is to say a commitment by which through a person's life one corresponds to a freely given gift and is thus open to transmitting it. In consonance with the constant teaching of the Church that procreation must have a pre-condition in marital love, Melina argues that artificial reproduction is an irresponsible form of generating human life because it takes place outside the marital love. He notes:

> Procreation that does not derive from authentic spousal love, and the corporeal and spiritual act that defines it, is not real responsible procreation. To defend the dignity of procreation of a human person there must be a real self-giving at his origins, both in the spiritual dimension and [free reciprocal self-giving in the conjugal context] and in the corporeal dimension.... detached from the context of conjugal love, a reproductive act loses the dignity of a procreation in which the spouses are collaborators with God in bringing forth of a new human life.[270]

Therefore, the magisterial methodological approach of *Donum Vitae* recognizes the role the couple play in procreation from the dimension of theology and morality, an approach that is basically anthropological.

1.5. On the Moral Object of the Simple Case IVF-ET

The basic problem in the Chapter Two is centered on the problem of the object of the human act. John Paul II in *Veritatis Splendor* has explained this problem and we shall do well to highlight some relevant teachings and commentaries of the document in this current section. Obviously, the

---

269 Ibid.
270 Ibid., 124. See also Ratzinger, "Uno sguardo teologico sulla procreazione umana," 507–521.

morality of the simple case IVF-ET cannot be evaluated adequately without the determination of the moral object of this procedure.[271] Among Catholic moral theologians, there exists a controversy on what constitutes the object that specifies the human act in its species or kind. St. Thomas Aquinas, whose thoughts are indispensable in this area, has not been unanimously understood among theologians with regards to his teaching on the object of the human act in which he indicates that the human act receives its species from its object.[272] This disagreement among Catholic moral theologians and ethicists influenced the contrasting views on the morality of the simple case IVF. As we know, procreation is a human act; it is an act freely and intentionally undertaken by the man and woman in a marital relationship as a consequence of their mutual self-gift of themselves.

Let us make recourse to the teaching of John Paul II in his encyclical *Veritatis Splendor* for classical insights into the morality of a human act. This document published on 6 August 6 1993 sought to treat fully and more deeply the issues touching the foundation of moral theology. One of such fundamental issues borders on the determination of the object of the moral act that had continued to be controversial among theologians and ethicists because of different theological methodologies or approaches employed. In fact, it has been attested by erudite scholars that *Veritatis Splendor* sets a hallmark of renewal in moral theology.[273] In this text, John Paul II exposes

---

271 On this point we do not intend to enter into the extensive philosophical discussions on the subject of human actions in general. Our focus is simply to underscore an aspect that serves our purpose in the context of our evaluation of the debates on the simple case IVF-ET by specifying the object of a human act according to what the Magisterium and some recent authors interpret Aquinas' teaching on this subject.

272 Duarte Sousa-Lara has presented a concise evaluation of contemporary interpretations of Aquinas on the object of a human act. He agrees that for Aquinas, the human act receives its species from the object of the act. However, he admits that this position remains controversial among commentators of Aquinas. Cf. Sousa-Lara, "Aquinas on the Object of the Human Act: A Reading in Light of the Texts and Commentators," in *Josephinum Journal of Theology* 15, 2 (2008): 243–276, at 244.

273 Cf. J. A. DiNoia and Romanus Cessario (eds.), *The Splendor of the Truth: Veritatis Splendor and the Renewal of Moral Theology* (Huntington: Our Sunday Visitor, 1999). This work undertaken by ten outstanding scholars,

some common theological trends (even among Catholic authors) that are erroneous in the evaluation of the morality of human actions. Those who follow the proportionalist and consequentialist approach to moral reasoning, claim that in order to qualify a concrete human action, either as being good or evil, one must take into account all the ends or goals for the sake of which a particular person decides to choose a particular course of action.[274] Some Catholic theologians who pursue these teleological theories of consequentialism and proportionalism, whose moral and ethical position John Paul II rejects as erroneous, nevertheless, have denied the representation of their views as presented in *Veritatis Splendor*. Although, the Pontiff did not specifically mention the identities of these moralists and ethicists, the common traits of their views are however articulated. In an article by William E. May in defense of *Veritatis Splendor*'s position on teleological theories of proportionalism and consequentialism, he traces the seminal development of these views to the so-called Majority Report of the Papal Commission for the Study of Population, the Family, and Nativity. Therein, he identifies the development of proportionalism in Catholic moral reasoning.[275] According to May, the proportionalists consider approach reveals, that the intention for a human act and a balance of the totality of the consequences of a chosen action should be calculated or established as to know whether the determinate behavior is the right or the wrong action to choose within given circumstances. The conclusion of this view would be that it is impossible to qualify as morally evil according to its species, its "object," the deliberate choice of certain kinds of behavior or specific acts, apart from a consideration of the intention for which the choice is made or the totality of the foreseeable consequences of that act for all persons concerned.[276] It can therefore be strongly suggested that this kind of reasoning

---

confirms the remarkable contribution of the Papal document in moral debate and the new approach in Moral Theology.

274 Cf. Peter Knauer, "Zu Grundbegriffen der Enzyklika 'Veritatis Splendor,'" in *Stimen der Zeit* 212 (1994): 14–26; Richard A. McCormick, "Some Early Reactions to *Veritatis Splendor*," in *Theological Studies* 55 (1994): 481–507.
275 Cf. William E. May, "John Paul II, Moral Theology, and Moral Theologians," in *The Splendor of the Truth*, 218–228.
276 *Veritatis Splendor*, n. 79.

pertains to the moral theories upon which the argument in support of the simple case is based.

In the contrary, the encyclical *Veritatis Splendor*, relying on the support of "intrinsically evil," that is, which are evil *always and per se*, on account of their object, and quite apart from the ulterior intentions of the one acting and the circumstances.[277] Expatiating on this point, John Paul II writes:

> The morality of the human act depends primarily and fundamentally on the "object" rationally chosen by the deliberate will as is borne out by the insightful analysis, still valid today, made by Saint Thomas. In order to be able to grasp the object of an act which specifies that act morally, it is therefore necessary to place oneself in the perspective of the acting person. The object of the act of willing is in fact a freely chosen kind of behaviour. To the extent that it is in conformity with the order of reason, it is the cause of the goodness of the will; it perfects us morally, and disposes us to recognize our ultimate end in the perfect good, primordial love. By the object of a given moral act, then, one cannot mean a process or an event of the merely physical order, to be assessed on the basis of its ability to bring about a given state of affairs in the outside world. Rather, that object is the proximate end of a deliberate decision which determines the act of willing on the part of the acting person.[278]

From the above citation, it would help to understand the proper teaching of the Church on the moral character of human actions and thereby reveals the error of those who contend the teaching on the existence of intrinsically evil acts in respect of determining the morality of a given choice of behavior. Once again, this is significant to evaluate the moral goodness or badness of the simple case as a means to generate human life. The Holy Father's teaching on the moral object, indicates that once the specified moral object of an act or chosen behavior is morally evil, there would be no point considering ulterior intentions of the acting person or the consequences that might result or the circumstances under which the act is to be achieved.

In order to further substantiate on the relevance of the moral object of an act, the text of the encyclical stresses this position using the following proposition:

---

277 Ibid., n. 80; Martin Rhonheimer, "Intrinsically Evil Acts and the Moral Viewpoint: Clarifying a Central Teaching of *Veritatis Splendor*," in *The Splendor of the Truth*, 161.
278 *Veritatis Splendor*, n. 78.

The primary and decisive element for moral judgment is the object of the human act, which establishes whether it is capable of being ordered to the good and to the ultimate end, which is God. This capability is grasped by reason in the very being of man, considered in his integral truth, and therefore in his natural inclinations, his motivations and his finalities, which always have a spiritual dimension as well. It is precisely these which are the contents of the natural law and hence that ordered complex of "personal goods" which serve the "good of the person": the good which is the person himself and his perfection. These are the goods safeguarded by the commandments, which, according to Saint Thomas, contain the whole natural law.[279]

Continuing on the path of clarification on the distinct moral significance of the object of a human act, John Paul II reiterates that:

If acts are intrinsically evil, a good intention or particular circumstances can diminish their evil, but they cannot remove it. They remain 'irremediably' evil acts; *per se* and in themselves they are not capable of being ordered to God and to the good of the person.... Consequently, circumstances or intentions can never transform an act intrinsically evil by virtue of its object into an act 'subjectively' good or defensible as a choice.[280]

Furthermore, the Catechism of the Church supports the above teaching when it states that: "it is an error to judge the morality of human acts by considering only the intention that inspires them or the circumstances (environment, social pressure, duress or emergency, etc.) which supply their context. [....]. One may not do evil so that good may result from it."[281]

On the whole, it must be admitted that the argument on the morality of the simple case IVF-ET is a complex one because it resides in the understanding of which factor determines the moral species of a human act. We believe that the classical method of moral reasoning, which bears witness to the teaching of John Paul II as expounded in *Veritatis Splendor*, lays claim to an adequate interpretation of Aquinas' understanding of the specification of the object of a human act. Adherents of this group of interpreters of Aquinas are distinguished from those who hold a physicalist and proportionalist interpretations of Aquinas' object of a human act. In the classical method of moral reasoning, the morality of a human act depends

---

279 *Veritatis Splendor*, n. 79. See also *Summa Theologiae*, I-II, q. 100, a. 1.
280 *Veritatis Splendor*, n. 81.
281 *Catechism of the Catholic Church*, n. 1756.

primarily and fundamentally on the object of the act. This group maintains that the other factors of a human act, namely, end and circumstances, are also important in the overall assessment of the morality of the act but only on the secondary level. This implies that if the moral value of the species of a human act is evil, that act, irrespective of other factors concerned, it cannot be a good act. It is within this perspective that those who support the rejection of the simple case IVF by the Magisterium base their argument.

For example, Rhonheimer's attempt to develop his argument in order to determine the object of the conjugal act reveals that:

> The so-called moral objects are the objects of the rationally guided will's choices to do something. Thus, the objects of human acts are neither the naturally given goals of inclinations [that is, natural ends] nor 'things' for which we are acting or aiming. Instead, they are, as Aquinas says, *'formae a ratione conceptae.'*[282]

This observation can be helpful to indicate that the object of the simple case IVF-ET or any other means of procreation is not the child as a consequence of the procedure or the intention of the couple to have a child. The object is the intentional content of the choice of the couple to use the simple case. The object of a human act in this situation refers to that which one does when one here and now chooses this procedure with an intention to have a child. Rhonheimer helps us to clarify this by stating that the object of the human act "is not about the foreseen outcome of the action seen as an event producing consequences, but about the chosen action itself in which the agent's will determines itself to a particular end which precisely shapes the action as a specific *kind* of action."[283] Would it then not be that the choice

---

282 Martin Rhonheimer, *Ethics of Human Procreation and the Defense of Human Life*: *Ethics of Procreation and the Defense of Human Life: Contraception, Artificial Fertilization, and Abortion*, Ed. William F. Murphy Jr. (Washington, D.C.: The Catholic University of America Press, 2010), 81. The internal reference from *Summa Theologica*, I-II, q. 18, a. 10: "*Species moralium actuum constituuntur ex formis, prout sunt a ratione conceptae.*" Rhonheimer understands this to mean that the species of the action is formed by the object of the act, which includes also the goal of the intention, which as well is a specifying object. Cf. Rhonheimer, Ibid., n19. See also William E. May, *Moral Absolutes, Catholic Tradition, Current Trends, and the Truth* (Milwaukee: Marquette University Press, 1989), 41–42.

283 Martin Rhonheimer, "Ethics of Norms and the Lost Virtues: Searching the Roots of Ethical Reasoning," in *Anthropotes* 9, 2 (1993): 238.

The Anthropological Argumentation of *Donum Vitae* 169

of this procedure is a decision that implies the "making" of a child and not a "begetting"? The couple that makes the choice of the IVF procedure may not think of the moral implications of their action as a "making" but their choice gives this meaning. Servais Pinckaers maintains a similar view in his contribution on the specification of the object of a human act. He admits that certainly, foreseeable results and consequences of actions are very important to assess the moral value of human actions, but they are secondary. For him, "the growing use of technology enables us to foresee results more clearly at social and even planetary levels. Nevertheless, this is not the primary element to be considered in the formation of a moral judgment."[284] Pinckaers cites *Veritatis Splendor* to affirm that the primary and fundamental determinant of the morality of a human act is the object rationally chosen by the deliberate will of the acting person.[285] The above position on the object of the act is in agreement with the classical tradition which interprets correctly the Aquinas' understanding of the object of the human act. Accepting the above analyses of Rhonheimer and Servais as a representation of this classical group of Catholic moral theologians and ethicists, inspired by the teaching of *Veritatis Splendor*, we would come to realize the error of the moral reasoning that denies the existence of intrinsically evil acts and the physicalistic and the consequentialist understanding of the object of a human act.[286] The moral doctrine on the existence of intrinsically evil acts is defended by the classical tradition as opposed to the other group.

Indeed, in the light of classical interpretation of Aquinas' texts on the object of the human act as seen in the foregoing, the moral object of the

---

284 Servais Pinckaers, "An Encyclical for the Future: *Veritatis Splendor*," in *The Splendor of the Truth*, 57.
285 Ibid. See also *Veritatis Splendor*, n. 78.1–2.
286 Martin Rhonheimer, "Intrinsically Evil Acts and the Moral Viewpoint: Clarifying a Central Teaching of *Veritatis Splendor*," in *The Splendor of the Truth*, 161–193. See also Rhonheimer, "Intentional Actions and the Meaning of Object: A Reply to Richard McCormick," in *The Splendor of the Truth*, 241–268; E. Colom and A. Rodríguez-Luño, *Scelti in Cristo per essere santi. Elementi di Teologia Morale Fondamentale*, Vol. 3 (Roma: Edizioni Università della Santa Croce, 2003), 194; Sousa-Lara, "Aquinas on the Object of the Human Act: A Reading in Light of the Texts and Commentators," 243–276.

simple case is considered an act of "making" a baby. In this view, the simple case implies "making" a child, but human life ought to be "begotten," received through a personal act of the couple's love, demonstrated in the union of body and spirit.[287] Since this is absent in the simple case, only the sperm and egg belong to them but it is not sufficient to procreate by the simple combination of the gamete cells of the spouses. In fact, it is claimed that the meaning implied in this procedure is not that of procreation but production. The medical personnel having received the sperm and the egg of the man and woman, supervises over the origin of the child in the laboratory using technical means, an action that is contrary to the dignity of the person because of the immediate and practical decisions and actions regarding the child's origin, undertaken by the medical personnel and not by the intimate act of love of his parents. This is true for the reason that all creation belongs to God, and he has designed how things should be in the world created by him, and for the fact that the generation of human life he has placed it within the context of marital relationship and much more as the fruit of a specific act of conjugal love. Therefore, the elimination of the bodily sexual union of the married man and woman in the generation of life goes contrary to God's plan and makes the means intrinsically wrong. The consequences of this manipulation of the order of human nature are signs of contempt for human life in its beginnings and a disregard for the means of its transmission. This can also change the image of marital union from an intimate union of love and life in the light of the Holy Trinity to triviality.

Furthermore, some moralists also believe that the moral quality of the simple case procedure cannot be derived from the totality of the conjugal life or from other conjugal acts before or after it. For instance, Chapelle underscores that the Instruction on the dignity of human procreation follows the moral doctrine that distinguishes the object from the intention or the circumstances.[288] It appears that the principle of totality which

---

287 Cf. May, "Catholic Teaching Concerning Homologous IVF," 86.
288 Chapelle, "The Dignity of Human Procreation," 67. The moral doctrine referenced in this case is in continuity with the teaching of Paul VI against contraception. "[....]. Neither is it valid to argue, as a justification for sexual intercourse which is deliberately contraceptive, that a lesser evil is to be preferred to a greater one, or that such intercourse would merge with procreative acts of past and future to form a single entity, and so be qualified by exactly

the dissenting theological opinion appeals to for the justification of the simple case IVF-ET, is not consistent with the best moral tradition as can be attested to in the discourses of Pius XII and in Paul VI's *Humanae Vitae*. This is precisely the moral tradition upon which *Donum Vitae*'s judgment on the simple case IVF-ET was conceived.[289]

Undoubtedly, those who are inclined to and indeed, hold the proportionalist and consequentialist views of moral reasoning are challenging the claim that the morality of a human act depends primarily on the object or species of the act. For these authors, to determine the morality of a concrete human action, the circumstances upon which the action occurs, the proximate as well as further intentions for which the action is undertaken must be taken account of. In this line of thought, there can be no classification of primary determining element of the moral value of a human action. McCormick has written extensively in defense of this theory and one of such impressive works challenging some aspects of *Veritatis Splendor* as well as Rhonheimer's article in support of the document's teaching on intrinsically evil acts.[290] The dissenting theological view of the Church's teaching on the simple case has not admitted the existence of intrinsically

---

the same moral goodness as these. Though it is true that sometimes it is lawful to tolerate a lesser moral evil in order to avoid a greater evil or in order to promote a greater good, it is never lawful, even for the gravest reasons, to do evil that good may come of it. In other words, to intend directly something which of its very nature contradicts the moral order, and which must therefore be judged unworthy of man, even though the intention is to protect or promote the welfare of an individual, of a family or of society in general. Consequently, it is a serious error to think that a whole married life of otherwise normal relations can justify sexual intercourse which is deliberately contraceptive and so intrinsically wrong." *Humanae Vitae*, n. 14.

289 On this, the Magisterium teaches that: "the question is asked whether the totality of the conjugal life in such situations is not sufficient to ensure the dignity proper to human procreation. It is acknowledged that IVF and ET certainly cannot supply for the absence of sexual relations, and cannot be preferred to the specific acts of conjugal union, given the risks involved for the child and the difficulties of the procedure." *Donum Vitae*, II, B/5.

290 Richard A. McCormick, "Some Early Reactions to *Veritatis Splendor*," in *Theological Studies* 55 (1994): 481–506. In response to McCormick's article, see Rhonheimer, "Intentional Actions and the Meaning of Object: A Reply to Richard McCormick," in *The Splendor of the Truth*, 241–268.

evil acts upon which the judgment on this procedure is derived; it accuses the Magisterium and her supporters of using deductive logic, which it claims to be erroneous on some moral issues.[291] From the Church's teaching, one can attest that there are certain realities that do not depend on time and case-by-case evaluation. It is sufficient to make a judgment based on its moral species inasmuch as it is about the human being having understood the nature of the person and of natural laws as well as indications from Revelation and the moral traditions of the Church.

However, the dissenting theologians do not agree with the classical interpretation of Aquinas' object of a human act. This disagreement has implications on their moral judgment of the simple case. For advocates of the simple case, the object of this procedure cannot be derived exclusively from the object of the technique apart from the intention of the couple and their circumstances. For these theologians, the object of a human act is specified by the totality of all the factors that pertain to the act. In their view, no one factor of an act is sufficient to render an act evil without a consideration of the intention and the circumstances related to the act. And so, the claim that the simple case is intrinsically evil cannot be taken for a good moral judgment to reject the simple case. Instead, they argue, the simple case IVF-ET can be a morally licit insofar as it promotes the marital relationship as well as grants the fulfillment of the couple with children in their marriage. This theological opinion proposes that the moral evaluation of the simple case should take into consideration all the elements of the act: its object, circumstances and end, in order to make a conclusion based on its result.[292] This position portrays the dissenting theologians as proposing the principle of proportionalism or consequentialism to justify the use of the simple case. In their view, the resort to the simple case is only a requirement to overcome and complement what nature lacks, such that even without the conjugal act and the seemingly intrusive nature of the procedure, the good of having a child can compensate for any defect in it.

From the foregoing, we can say that the dissenting theologians would be getting it incomplete to emphasize only the good intention or circumstances

---

291 Cf. Hunt, "New Vatican Instruction on Human Life and Procreation," 245.
292 Cf. McCormick, *Notes on Moral Theology*, 118.

The Anthropological Argumentation of *Donum Vitae* 173

of the couple as sufficient factors for moral acceptability of the simple case and not the species of the act or the meaning implied in the act of generating human life without the conjugal act. The teaching of *Veritatis Splendor* is illuminating here:

> The doctrine of the object as a source of morality represents an authentic explication of the Biblical morality of the Covenant and of the commandments, of charity and of the virtues. The moral quality of human acting is dependent on this fidelity to the commandments, as an expression of obedience and of love. For this reason – we repeat – the opinion must be rejected as erroneous which maintains that it is impossible to qualify as morally evil according to its species the deliberate choice of certain kinds of behavior or specific acts, without taking into account the intention for which the choice was made or the totality of the foreseeable consequences of that act for all persons concerned. Without the rational determination of the morality of human acting as stated above, it would be impossible to affirm the existence of an 'objective moral order' and to establish any particular norm the content of which would be binding without exception. This would be to the detriment of human fraternity and the truth about the good, and would be injurious to ecclesial communion as well.[293]

The object of a human act as we tried to state above, encompasses both the spiritual and physical aspects of the action corresponding to the nature of man as a composite being of body and spirit; as such, this act is conceived, as the consequence of a deliberate will. Human procreation in a morally acceptable way embraces essentially the bodily and spiritual union of the man and woman. Both the unitive and procreative aspects of this act of conjugality constitute a whole action in such a way that it is possible to talk of procreation as having a single object. Hence, it would be morally wrong to choose one aspect, say the procreative while neglecting the unitive or vice versa. No doubt, in a certain sense, we can talk of human procreation with a series of connected meanings and objects; these have significance only as components of the entire act of procreation. So, it is a kind of organized system from both biological and moral dimensions. In fact, "procreation is effectuated by loving, mutual self-giving of the spouses in the totality of their body-spirit-unity. Therefore, every procreative act actually is expressing loving union; human life arises from this love between a man and a woman."[294] Even if their act of bodily and spiritual

---

293 *Veritatis Splendor*, n. 82.
294 Rhonheimer, *Ethics of Procreation and the Defense of Human Life*, 83.

union does not achieve its natural function in a new human life, because the intentional action corresponds to the means (conjugal act) ordered to the generation of life, the act would still have a procreative meaning as its inherent consequence. But, the moral object of the simple case IVF-ET procedure is different, because the generation of human life without the sexual act is implicitly, as we said before, a type of "making" and not a "doing" to achieve procreation.

1.6. Summary

The foundation of the Church's teaching on artificial procreation is the human person who stands in a relationship with God and through whom God makes possible the generation of new human life. Human procreation is not a chance event but a love event of God extending his love to the spouses to collaborate with him in the work of creation. God re-enacts his creative act in each new life that is brought forth. Human procreation is both a biological and spiritual act corresponding to the nature of the persons as composite beings of body and soul. From another aspect, it is both a divine and human project. The implication of this requires that in intervening in the transmission of new human life, it is not simply the biological aspect that is involved but the spiritual as well. The spiritual corresponds to the divine pole and the biological has its natural order but there can be no separation between these two dimensions.

Fundamentally, the logic of *Donum Vitae* takes its force from the nature of the person and from the unity of persons in marriage. The insight from this methodology has implications in the light of the dignity of human life as a gift of God taking into consideration its origins, development and ultimate destiny. Therefore, the mode of transmission of human life should respect the immensity of his absolute worth, the context of his generation and the divine moral laws that regulate his being and actions. In view of these dimensions, the Instruction's conclusion on the simple case IVF and similar techniques cannot be said to be inadequate, biologically based and misplaced.

B. The Dignity of Human Procreation

1.1. An Overview of the Argument on the Dignity of Human Procreation

The dignity of human procreation is derived from the dignity of the person. Anthropologically, man is radically unique and unrepeatable and possesses an interiority that distinguishes him from other created beings. Besides, theologically, man stands in a unique relationship with God for he is the only being created by God for himself. Therefore, the generation of human life acquires a special meaning due to the profundity of his being. And so, the child's coming into being is willed by God to be the fruit of love of his parents situated in the conjugal act. The Church teaches that for procreation to correspond to the dignity of the person the whole process must begin in the conjugal act and fertilization must not be reduced to an act of producing or making as it is the case with IVF. The Catholic moral doctrine on the conjugal act has been affirmed and defended as well as dissented from and criticized by some theologians. The debate on the moral acceptability of the simple case IVF-ET largely rests on the teaching that procreation must not be separated from the embrace of bodily union of the couple. This section is dedicated to the theological opinion that affirms, defends and supports the magisterial understanding of the conjugal act upon which the simple case is prohibited as a morally wrong means of human procreation.[295] The conjugal act is believed to be the only source and origin of the new human life. It is in the conjugal act that God creates anew human life. The conjugal act bears testimony to God's contact with man and woman for the

---

295 For a comprehensive bibliographical study on the conjugal act, see the works of: Janet E. Smith, *"Humanae Vitae," a Generation Later* (Washington, D.C.: Catholic University of America Press, 1993); Janet E. Smith (ed.), *Why Humanae Vitae Was Right: A Reader* (San Francisco: Ignatius Press, 1993); Alain Mattheeuws, *Union et procreation* (Paris: Les Editions du Cerf, 1989); Carlo Caffarra, *Etica generale della sessualità* (Milano: Ares, 1992); Donald P. Asci, *The Conjugal Act as a Personal Act: A Study of the Catholic Concept of the Conjugal Act in the Light of Christian Anthropology* (San Francisco: Ignatius Press, 2002); William E. May, Ronald Lawler and Joseph Boyle, Jr., *Catholic Sexual Ethics: A Summary, Explanation and Defense*, 3rd edition (Huntington, IN: Our Sunday Visitor Inc., 2011).

continuity of the human race. The conjugal act expresses the unity of the couple in their bodily and spiritual dimensions, the unity which is a symbol of their mutual self donation and reception. It is within this context and in this event that God the author of life, grants the gift of new life as a fruit of love, first between the spouses and with him. Therefore, the "special nature of the transmission of human life in marriage" is clearly and understandably different from the transmission of life in other animals. It is intentional, calculative, purposive and governed by laws, the laws of God "inscribed in the very being of man and woman." The laws considered here are the natural laws and not some mechanical or even simply biological laws. These are the perspectives that we are considering below.

1.2. The Unitive-Procreative Significance of the Conjugal Act

Certainly, the Vatican Instruction *Donum Vitae* in a certain sense is adjudged to be the first magisterial document to expound on the essence of the conjugal act in respect of the two meanings or significance connected in that marital act and to apply it in a rigorous manner to artificial reproductive technologies. No doubt, previous magisterial documents dealing on the subject of marriage had offered deep and profound theological insights that are still relevant.[296] For instance, *Humanae Vitae*'s exposition of the principle of inseparability of the conjugal act is remarkable and innovative. And so, when *Donum Vitae* recaptures this teaching and specifically applies it to artificial procreation, and in so doing the Church reiterates its doctrine regarding the truth about the unity of marriage and *ipso facto* emphasizes the moral obligation that is anthropologically and theologically significant in the decision to procreate.[297] The prohibition of the simple case IVF and

---

[296] Cf. Pius XI, *Casti Connubii*, 1930; Pius XII, *Discourse to the Fourth International Congress of Catholic Doctors*; 1949; Second Vatican Council: *Gaudium et Spes*, 1965; Paul VI, *Humanae Vitae*, 1968 and John Paul II, *Familiaris Consortio*, 1983.

[297] Cf. *Donum Vitae*, II, B/4, a; *Humanae Vitae*, n. 12. In *Humanae Vitae*, we read that: "Huiusmodi doctrina, quae ab Ecclesiae Magisterio saepe exposita est, in nexu indissolubili nititur, a Deo statuto, quem homini sua sponte infringere non licet, inter significationem unitatis et significationem procreationis, quae ambae in actu coniugali insunt. Etenim propter intimam suam rationem, coniugii actus, dum maritum et uxorem artissimo sociat vinculo, eos idoneos

other forms of artificial procreation hinges on this principle of inseparability and by extension the indignity and contempt associated with external fertilization of human embryo. The Instruction actually acknowledges the fact that the simple case is not marked by ethical negativity found in extra-conjugal procreation, but on the basis that it deprives human procreation of the dignity that is proper and connatural to it, this procedure remains unacceptable on moral grounds.[298] However, some authors still argue that this principle, even if considered applicable to contraception, would only be improperly applied to artificial procreation because the principle in itself does not indicate that procreation should not take place without the sexual intercourse.[299] This view can be illuminated by the text of *Donum Vitae* itself when it states that the moral value of the intimate link between the goods of marriage and between the meanings of the conjugal act is based upon the unity of the human being, a unity involving body and spiritual soul. Spouses mutually express their personal love in the "language of the body," which clearly involves both "spousal meanings" and parental ones. The conjugal act by which spouses mutually express their self-gift and at the same time express openness to the greater gift, which is new human life. It is an act that is inseparably corporal and spiritual. It is in their bodies and through their bodies that the spouses consummate their marriage and are able to become father and mother.[300]

---

etiam facit ad novam vitam gignendam, secundum leges in ipsa viri et mulieris natura inscriptas. Quodsi utraque eius- modi essentialis ratio, unitatis videlicet et procreationis, ser- vatur, usus matrimonii sensum mutui verique amoris suumque ordinem ad celsissimum paternitatis munus omnino retinet, ad quod homo vocatur."

298 Cf. *Donum Vitae*, II, B/5. The dignity of human procreation that is deprived by the simple case cannot easily pointed out except through reflection on the value of human life and the consequences implied in such a technique. It becomes even more complicated is this procedure were to commence after an intercourse supervised by a technician who waits to harvest the sperm deposited in the vagina. The role of the technician would be questionable and the nature and meaning of the procedure of IVF vis-à-vis the human life being conceived outside the womb.

299 This dissenting opinion has already been treated in chapter two of this work.

300 *Donum Vitae*, II, B/4, b.

Furthermore, in order to respect the "language of their bodies" and their natural generosity, the conjugal union must take place with respect for its openness to procreation; and the procreation of a person must be the fruit and the result of married love. This married love has its summit in the conjugal act, the symbol of their unreserved self-donation and reception of themselves. Thus, the origin of the human being is 'linked to the union, not only biological but also spiritual, of the parents, made one by the bond of marriage.' In respect of this, "fertilization achieved outside the bodies of the couple remains by this very fact deprived of the meanings and the values which are expressed in the 'language of the body' and in the union of human persons."[301] The just cited paragraph of the Instruction captures succinctly the essential elements of the magisterial teaching position on artificial procreation. The significance of the two ends of the conjugal act are seen in the light of the nature of the human person as a composite creature of body and soul. This statement equally clarifies and applies the principle to clearly suggest that human procreation can only be the causal effect of the marital sexual act as an expression of the mutual self-gift and reception of the spouses. In other words, procreation may not be sought outside the conjugal act as a personal act that is inseparably corporal and spiritual and essentially unitive of the couple.

A systematic argument to show the reasonableness in the use of the principle of inseparability to prohibit contraception and artificial procreation has equally been marshaled out by Rhonheimer.[302] He likens this principle to the substantial unity of man and insists that there is an essential unity between love and procreation. He sees procreation as a basic human good to the same extent as is human life. He therefore proposes two elements that can be useful to clarify this principle: human procreation presupposes spiritual love and insofar as it is love between human beings of male and female sexes, possesses procreative dimension by virtue of its inclination to consummation in bodily dimension. The second element seems to speak more clearly in terms of substantiating the reason for the inseparability principle and here we can refer to the author more directly:

---

301 Ibid.
302 Rhonheimer, *Ethics of Procreation and the Defense of Human Life*, 71–227.

> Love between male and female, insofar as it tends, by its very nature, toward consummation in bodily union – that is, insofar as it springs from the *naturalis inclinatio ad coniunctionem maris et feminae*, from sexual inclination – possesses a procreative dimension, because it is love between two bodily – constituted spiritual beings. In other words, the loving bodily union of male and female is, by its own nature, 'service to transmission of life.'... Therefore, the 'inseparable connection' of the two meanings signifies their *reciprocal inclusive correlation*. The bodily reality of procreation receives its fully human specification from spiritual love; the spiritual love of the married persons receives its specification as a determinate *sort* of love from the procreative function of the body. Thus for a correct and exhaustive understanding of the inseparability principle, it is decisive to recognize that these two meanings neither merely 'added' to each other, nor merely conjoined or accumulated 'functions' of which each has its full intelligibility *independently* from the other. Rather, each receives its full intelligibility as a *human* reality – its fully *human* meaning – precisely *from the other*. Procreation considered independently from spiritual love *is no longer the same thing*.... This precisely is what follows from man's substantial body-spirit unity.[303]

Rhonheimer's submission is quite compelling because of the indication that the meaning or relevance of each of the two dimensions of the conjugal act receives its reasonableness with reference to the other dimension. This for him is based on the structural and functional reality of the human being. In fact, he gives the impression that any procreative procedure such as the simple case IVF that excludes the sexual intercourse of the couple has a different meaning and contradicts the moral requirement of human procreation. Hence,

> If we consider things in this perspective of substantial unity of body and spirit, then the reason why these two meanings are inseparably connected becomes obvious: by separating them we would alter both the meaning of human procreation and the meaning of marital loving union. Both meanings are not extrinsically, but intrinsically connected: the very connection constitutes the specifically human content of both meanings. And, the horizon within which this link is understood is the corporeal-spiritual composition of the human person.[304]

Furthermore, the conjugal act is equally believed to be the most personal and non – transferable act of the spouses. While this act unites the couple in mutual love and marital friendship, it achieves its finality in procreation. In other words, procreation results as the natural consequence of the sexual

---

303 Ibid., 77.
304 Ibid., 78.

act. It can also be manipulated to result outside the normal context but this constitutes an aberration on the moral plane. This idea finds its better explanation by Ratzinger when he sustains that:

> Conjugal sexuality is the expression of the definitive gift that the spouse makes of himself to the other, and as such confirms and aids in the spouses a communion of total and indissoluble love. It is because of this, its intimate truth, that conjugal sexuality, precisely in the specific conjugal act of the spouses' union, is called to a *participationem specialem quondam in suiipsius opera creative* [namely, God's] [...]. It is therefore neither by chance nor by human decision that these two fundamental meanings – the unitive and the procreative – reside in the conjugal act. This 'cohabitation,' or connection, is a moral requirement based on the very nature of man and on his relationship with God the Creator. It is an onto-axiological requirement.[305]

This means that the two dimensions or values of the conjugal act may not be separated owing to the fact that: (1) they are ontologically structured accordingly; (2) they form the basic goods of marriage and in these goods marriage finds its purpose; and (3) God manifests his love for man and continues his work of creation within the context of marriage in the conjugal act. There is therefore, an intrinsic coherence in the structure of the conjugal act, such that within this structure, admirable and internal harmony that befits the dignity of the person and of procreation is required. In this consists the dignity of human procreation.

On the strength of the Church's teaching, the conjugal act as an essential expression of marriage has a theological foundation since marriage is as

---

305 Ratzinger, "Preface," in *Instruction Donum Vitae: Commentaries and Studies*, viii. The internal reference comes from the document Pastoral Constitution *Gaudium et Spes*, n. 50. John Paul II had several times in different occasions, taught that in procreation God's intervention as the Creator cannot be refuted. He states, "at the beginning of every human life there is the creative act of God: no man comes into existence by chance; he is always the end of God's creative love. It follows from the essential truth of faith and reason that the capacity for procreation, inscribed in human sexuality, is in its deepest truth a cooperation with the creative power of God. It also follows that man and woman are not the arbiters of the same capacity, nor are they masters, since they are called in it and through it to be participants of God's creative decision." John Paul II, *Address to Priests Participating in the Study Seminar on Responsible Procreation*, 17 September 1983, in *Insegnamenti di Giovanni Paolo II*, 6.2:561–561–564. Cited in Sgreccia, *Personalist Bioethics*, 396.

well a divine institution. In *Casti Connubii*, Pius XI teaches that marriage is not a human invention but that marriage has its origin in God. Man and woman out of love and free will, exchange their consents to be husband and wife in response to God's plan of creation in order to be in a communion of love and life for the rest of their life on earth.[306] Therefore, God has designed that marriage be oriented naturally towards several values that are inherently connected. With reference to the teaching of St. Augustine, Pius XI names these values or goods to be children (*bonum prolis*), fidelity (*bonum fidei*) and sacrament (*bonum sacramenti*).[307] The Second Vatican Council also highlights the fact that God established marriage. The document *Gaudium et Spes* describes marriage as:

> The intimate partnership of married life and love has been established by the Creator and qualified by His laws, and is rooted in the conjugal covenant of irrevocable personal consent... By their very nature, the institution of matrimony itself and conjugal love is ordained for the procreation and education of children, and find in them their ultimate crown.[308]

We can say the most important elements in this description are: first, God established the institution of marriage; second, marriage is a partnership of life and love and is ordered to the generation of new life. Hence, it affirms the truth that procreation is limited to marriage by God.

In defending the principle of inseparability of the two meanings of the conjugal act, another perspective is expressed by May. He articulates that the bond between the unitive and procreative ends of the conjugal act is properly marriage. In other words, the purpose of marriage lies in the unity of these two ends. These are the goods of marriage. He explains:

> The marital act, in other words, is by its own inner nature love-giving or unitive and opens to the transmission of human life or procreative. And it is so precisely because it is marital, i.e., an act participating in marriage and the goods perfective of it. The bond, therefore, that unites the two meanings of the marital act is the marriage itself. But, 'what God has joined together, let no man put asunder.' It is for this reason, I believe that there is an 'unbreakable connection between the unitive meaning and the procreative meaning' of the conjugal act.[309]

---

306 Cf. Pius XI, *Casti Connubii*, nn. 6–7.
307 Ibid., n. 10.
308 *Gaudium et Spes*, n. 48.
309 May, *Marriage*, 84.

By this assertion, May finds fault with the use of IVF and even the so-called simple case because this technique separates or put asunder to the unity between the love-union and the procreative aspects of the conjugal act. Hence, at least, the voluntary separation of procreation from the sexual act, contradicts both the natural principle which indicates that procreation flows from the sexual act and the moral-theological prescription that human procreation is distinctively a human act which collaborates with God's act of creation in a manner that befits the human being to be born and the ones who are co-creators with God.

Furthermore, May argues that the generation of human life outside the specific conjugal act is a violation of the will of God that only the marital act is suitable for such a noble mission. In taking this view, he makes reference to Pius XII's discourse that:

> We must never forget this: It is only the procreation of a new life according to the will and plan of the Creator which brings with it – to an astonishing degree of perfection – the realization of the desired ends. This is, at the same time, in harmony with the dignity of the marriage partners, with their bodily and spiritual natures, and with the normal and happy development of the child.[310]

May proposes another argument that the simple case is not a marital act. This argument advanced by May against the simple case indicates that only the marital act is worthy of being the source of human life, and because the simple case is a non-marital act, it is therefore not worthy of human life. May argues:

> It is obvious that heterologous insemination/fertilization and cloning are 'non-marital.' But 'non-marital' too are homologous artificial insemination and IVF. Even though married persons have collaborated in these procedures and even those procedures make use of gamete cells supplied by husband and wife, the procedures are 'non-marital' because the marital status of the man and the woman participating in them is accidental and not essential.[311]

May's assumption suggests that human procreation is a personal and exclusive act legitimately performed by persons who are in an exclusive marital

---

310 Pius XII, *Discourse at the Fourth International Congress of Medical Doctors*. Cited in May, "Catholic Teaching on the Laboratory Generation of Human Life," in *The Gift of Life*, 79–80.
311 May, *Catholic Bioethics and the Gift of Human Life*, 86.

union. This personal act is irreplaceable and non-substitutable, hence the use of IVF that implies the actions and involvement of third parties in the most intimate marital union makes it a non-marital act and therefore morally wrong. Applying non-marital to the simple case IVF indicates that the procedure bears the picture of a delegable role and not an irreplaceable personal act that is marital. This is so in the sense that the role of the technician or the technique does not essentially pertain to the marital union of the spouses.

1.3. The Conjugal Act: Its Unity and Plenitude

The conjugal act has its unity and fullness. Elio Sgreccia hits on this very point that many scholars including Catholic who have sympathy for the hypothetic technique called simple case IVF seem to overlook. It precisely resides in the relationship between the human body and the conjugal act. The Church teaches that human conception outside the bodies of the couple remains by this very fact incomplete of the meanings and values that are expressed in the "language of the body" and in the union of human persons. The human body in its natural design has the power of communicating love by virtue of being male or female.[312] In the light of this, Sgreccia sustains that an act of procreation without bodily expression deprives this act not only of its biological factor, but also of the personal communion that can be expressed only through the body in its plenitude and unity.[313] Hence, the substitution of the bodily act with technology is a reduction of the conjugal act, a kind of disruption in the harmony of procreation and this is morally problematic. For Sgreccia, this kind of degradation of the conjugal act to a sort of technical act is pernicious to human dignity and the process of procreation. He therefore supports the judgment of the Instruction on the simple case IVF by stating that:

> Among all the expressive acts or languages of the body, the conjugal act is the one that has the characteristic of plenitude and totality: to reduce procreation to a technological fact, therefore, means to establish a relationship of domination, 'producer subject – produced object'; it also means to degrade and impoverish the procreative act from both a theological and an anthropological point of view.[314]

---

312 *Donum Vitae*, II, B/4, b.
313 Sgreccia, "Moral Theology and Artificial Procreation," in *Gift of Life*, 132.
314 Ibid.

Sgreccia strongly believes that the judgment of the Magisterium on the simple case is not too strict or rigid but adequate. This is in view of protecting the dignity of the human person and the means of procreation considering that the conjugal act expresses the unity and plenitude of human procreation and of the dignity of every human being. Indeed, a procreative act that is devoid of full personal and bodily communion would be less than human procreation. In his conversation with the Catholic News Agency, Sgreccia among other things gave the indication that in extracorporeal fertilization, the unitive dimension of the spouses, expressed through the gift of self in the conjugal act is missing.[315] We can deduce from his thoughts as noted above, that because the simple case IVF lacks the essential personal dimension required in human procreation, it is morally defective and unworthy of man.

An appeal to the axiological structure of human sexuality is equally attested to in the argument against artificial procreation that seeks procreation outside the conjugal act of which the simple case is a case in point. For instance, the analysis of the anthropology and axiology of human sexuality is well treated by Rodríguez-Luño.[316] In the treatment of this matter, Rodríguez-Luño expounds the two dimensions which sexuality by God's design is meant for. He argues that the demands of conjugal communion are open to those of procreation. Yet, the demands of procreation are equally open to those of conjugal communion in a sense that the children also strengthen the bond of marriage. Here, one sees the plenitude and significance of the conjugal act, such that the voluntary dissolution of these dimensions naturally contradicts and injures the value of this sacred activity and relationship. This injury may not be so evident outside a wider vision of human anthropology. However, it has moral consequences in connection with the meaning and values of conjugal union.

Again, another theologian, Nicholas Tonti-Filippini assumes that even if sexual intercourse were to be performed by the couple in the simple case IVF, it would still fall short of the moral requisite for the dignity of human procreation. His concern is based on the assumption, that should

---

315 Ibid., *A Conversation with the Catholic News Agency*, 24 April 2006, Vatican City.
316 Rodríguez-Luño, *Scelti in Cristo per Essere Santi*, 345–359.

this procedure occur in the context of sexual intercourse, there would be need for a physician to monitor or guide the procreative process in order to harvest the sperm for onward laboratory work. Regarding this hypothesis, Tonti-Filippini observes,

> ... there is a moral question which must be answered concerning the licitness of the conjugal act being performed on cue, so to speak, so that sperm can be harvested immediately. The conjugal act in those circumstances would be a generative act, perhaps, but the clinical control required and the lack of spontaneity would reduce, if not totally exclude, the unitive expression of love. The conjugal act would be reduced to merely a mechanical method of obtaining sperm.[317]

Therefore, in the simple case IVF the plenitude of the conjugal act is distorted by the intrusion of the physician and this constitutes rather a moral problem. The action of the physician towards achieving fertilization outside the womb following the manipulated or supervised sexual intercourse remains a more dominant role than that of the couple. In other words, the role of the couple is subservient or secondary to the one performed by the technician, indeed, fertilization can be seen as the result of the medical intervention or even the consequence of the handwork of professionalism rather than the fruit of the couple's marital act.

Along the same line of thought on the assumption indicated by Tonti-Filippini that the simple case IVF could involve the sexual act though monitored, Josef Seifert has offered a philosophical approach to this question. Against the claim of the supporters of the simple case IVF that this procedure is "assistance" to the conjugal act, Seifert's observation points to the contrary. The central point around which he weaves his argument against artificial procreation relates to the principle of *causal continuity*. This entails that the conjugal act must be the principal cause of fertilization and there must be a natural continuity of motion initiated by the sexual act. And so, "assistance to the conjugal act can be defined as an activity which respects the meaningful and non-substitutable bond between the personal

---

317 Nicholas Tonti-Filippini, "IVF: The Role of the Technician," in Charles Connolly (ed.), *New Life: Catholic Teaching on Technology and Fertilization, with Commentaries* (Dublin: Four Courts Press, 1987), 71–72.

conjugal act and procreation as its effect."[318] Seifert indicates in his critical essay some relevant criteria for judgment: continuity and unity. In his view, it seems clear that the most basic requirement for the correct application of the term "assistance" or help to any act – rather than speaking of substitution – is that a certain effect proceeds from the act as from its cause in such a way that we can speak of a continuity of the process which leads from the cause to the effect. He claims that the conjugal act up until fertilization is achieved in order to ascertain that the medical procedure does not replace the conjugal act.

To substantiate his claim, Seifert has offered a phenomenal view on the fundamental distinction between replacement of the conjugal act and assistance to it. According to him,

> Such a "continuity" of the causal process, in its turn, can situate itself on two levels: on that of the mere natural causality and on that of the personal act that gives rise to something. And on each level it can involve a temporal continuity or a "logical unity" of the causal process itself or both. The two orders, that of the natural causality and that of the personal acts, are most intimately intertwined in the mode in which the conjugal act gives rise to procreation. For of course, it is not the personal act as such which leads to procreation, but all kinds of physiological processes which are distinct from the personal act of conjugal union but in part flow from it [...], and which continue to follow that conjugal act hours and days after its consummation, and which in part are simply produced by the various physiological processes inside the bodies of the spouses.[319]

It could be discerned from Seifert's submission that the medical intervention in order to be truly licit, must neither frustrate the natural process after normal sexual intercourse between the couple nor introduce what is essentially strange to the process. This means that the intervention should not constitute a significant or principal part of the process but rather be subservient to the process. Seifert would therefore defend the conclusion of the Magisterium that the simple case is not a licit means of procreation because it lacks the unity and plenitude of the values needed in human

---

318 Josef Seifert, "Substitution of the Conjugal Act or Assistance to It?" IVF, GIFT and Some Other Medical Interventions, Philosophical Reflections on the Vatican Declaration *Donum Vitae*," in *Anthropotes* 4 (1988): 274.
319 Ibid.

procreation because the procedure itself replaces the conjugal act that is required in human procreation.

1.4. The Conjugal Act: A Personal Act of the Couple

To say the conjugal act is a personal act indicates that it pertains to and incorporates the qualifying characteristics of the action of the human person. But, however, it refers to the intimate action of the spouses by virtue of their personhood. This goes far to signify on the one hand that this act is only performed by human beings and *ipso facto* carries with it moral consequences. It can be said, "the conjugal act is the type of activity that only human persons can engage in because it relies upon specifically human traits in its very performance."[320] The conjugal act is specifically a unique type of human act and its uniqueness comes from the truth of marriage between a man and woman, an interpersonal form of human relationship.[321] On this ground, the conjugal act becomes an irreplaceable and non-transferable act exclusive to a man and a woman in a particular marital union. By means of the marital act, the spouses make manifest the consent they had made on their wedding to donate and receive each other as husband and wife in an enduring life-long communion of life and love. The conjugal act expresses and perfects the couple's love for each other and

---

320 Asci, *The Conjugal Act as a Personal Act*, 273.
321 This reflects the teaching of John Paul II particularly on his personalist understanding of marriage. In *Familiaris Consortio*, n. 3, one reads the indication of the fact of marriage or the conjugal act being a personal act, by which spouses give and receive themselves and await the reality of child as gift. In fact he locates procreation only within the personal love between husband and wife and a child as the supreme gift of their own mutual gift of themselves. "In its most profound reality, love is essentially a gift; and conjugal love, while leading the spouses to the reciprocal 'knowledge' which makes them 'one flesh,' does not end with the couple, because it makes them capable of the greatest possible gift, the gift by which they become cooperators with God for the giving life to a new human person. Thus the couple, while giving themselves to one another, give not just themselves but also the reality of children, who are a living reflection of their love, a permanent sign of conjugal unity and a living and inseparable synthesis of their being a father and a mother."

helps them participate in the goods of marriage and the consummation of their marriage.[322]

Expressing his view on the personal nature of the conjugal act, Cormac Burke indicates that the uniqueness of this act is not derived from the fact of sharing sensation between the spouses but the sharing of power. By power he means:

> An extraordinary life-related, creative, physical, sexual power…. Other physical expressions of affection do not go beyond the level of mere gesture; they remain a symbol of union desired. But the conjugal act is not a mere symbol. In marital intercourse, something real has been exchanged, with full gift and acceptance of conjugal masculinity and femininity.[323]

The power so referred to here, is based on the fact that the spouses are married to each other and the act of conjugality is so performed in view of its natural consequence. This explains why even if one of the spouses specializes in artificial procreative procedure, they cannot claim to use the same power to intervene in their marital relationship to achieve procreation. The technical power is different from the conjugal power and do operate at different levels in life. Indeed, the technical power does not pertain to marital union and it cannot be marital. Hence, it would amount to a transfer of a non – transferable personal power and right, understood in the moral sense for the couple to mix up these "powers" in a bid to avoid a third person entering their marital intimacy. May, an erudite defender of the *Donum Vitae*'s conclusion on the simple case IVF writes,

> The marital act considered precisely as a human, personal act, is more than a genital act between a man and a woman who simply happen to be married. It is an act that inwardly participates in the their one-flesh, marital union and in the 'goods' or 'blessings' of marriage… the goods of loving fidelity and children. The *marital act*, therefore, as distinct from a merely *genital act*, is one that is (1) open to the communication of spousal love and (2) open to God's gift of human life.[324]

These observations by Burke and May suggest that the conjugal act being a personal act is not concerned with the couple's sharing of a function or

---

322 Cf. *Code of Cannon Law*, Can. 1061 § 1.
323 Cormac Burke, *Covenanted Happiness* (Princeton: Scepter Press, 1999), 91.
324 William E. May, "Anthropological Advances in *Humanae Vitae*," in *Humanae vitae: servizio profetico per l'uomo* (Rome: Editrice Ave, 1995), 379.

The Dignity of Human Procreation 189

a satisfaction reserved for them, but a sharing of themselves as human persons.

To further buttress the claim that the simple case IVF-ET is illicit, Melina observes that IVF destroys the personal dimension in human procreation. In fact,

> In reality, when artifice is introduced into the spring of life, to the point of replacing the very personal action of the corporeal and spiritual union of the parents, there is a deformation of the dignity of procreating and obscuring of the presence of God in the origins of the personal subject.[325]

In his well-reasoned excursus, Melina sustains that when human procreation is left for biomedical science to replace the specifically personal act, the dignity of the person is undermined. In other words, artificial procreation like the simple case IVF cannot be judged based on the technical efficiency of the procedure but on its moral validity. This explains away the Instruction's principle that the techniques of artificial procreation must not be evaluated based on their technical efficiency but in relation to the dignity of the person and conjugal union. It is necessary to be conscious of the personal dimensions that determine the ethical substance of the act. Melina believes that the conjugal act is a personal act and must therefore not be substituted by technical efficiency. If this is omitted, it becomes the vector of a logic that deforms the human beyond the original intentions that motivated it.[326] This observation of Melina is a caution on the extent in which biomedical science can assist in human procreation otherwise it usurps the responsibility of the personal aspect of procreation which is morally unacceptable. In this perspective, he gives the impression that the simple case IVF procedure replaces the personal dimension that is the principal factor in human procreation.

Another interesting point of view that is raised against the simple case IVF can be seen in the thoughts of Tonti-Filippini.[327] He focuses his argument on the role of the technician in the simple case IVF. He notes that the technician practically constitutes a third party and an intruder in the

---

325 Melina, "The Intrinsic Logic of Interventions in the Field of Human Artificial Procreation: Ethical Aspects," 436.
326 Ibid.
327 Tonti-Filippini, "IVF: The Role of the Technician," in *New Life*, 71–74.

intimacy of couple's marital act. Secondly, he thinks that role of the technician has a moral implication and precisely that the technician dispenses with or usurps the responsibility of the spouses, namely, that of being the initiators and source of fertilization of the new life through the conjugal act. Tonti-Filippini observes:

> IVF, in even the simplest case, would involve a significant intrusion into the conjugal relationship by the IVF technician. The choice is made with the good motive of assisting the couple to have a child which they would not otherwise have, but it involves the technician intruding into the sexual intimacy of the couple by having them perform the conjugal act on cue, but more than that, the technician stands in as 'parent' to the child in the former's acts of initiating the life and of custodianship for the time that it takes the embryo to mature sufficiently so that implantation can take place. An objective analysis of the technician's role must therefore see him or her as displacing the role of the parents in the initial stage of the new life.[328]

In the light of the above submission, Tonti-Filippini indicates that the physician or technician has not merely assisted the couple in the process of procreation but stands in a special and novel relationship to the child who develops. Indeed, the technician makes himself to be an active agent who could claim responsibility for the child's coming into being. The involvement of an active external party to achieve human fertilization has also been criticized by Charles Connolly as one of the reasons for the moral illicitness of homologous IVF-ET and even in the simple case. He notes that this procedure is morally illicit because it is achieved outside the body of the couple and more so through the actions of third parties and thus the generation of the child as an act of procreation is deprived of its proper perfection. The proper perfection is said to be allowing the child to be the fruit of a loving conjugal act of the spouses' cooperation with God. For him the simple case IVF-ET is not allowed for the generation of a child because the child would not be received as the fruit of a normal conjugal act.[329] No doubt, it

---

328 Ibid., 72. The author goes on to indicate that although the physician takes the function of the child's parents but he/she lacks the love of parents and without this love, the child is considered by the physician as an object. Hence, at this initial stage, the "embryo is more the object of a making than a consequence of love-making and is not an equal third party to the expression of love." Ibid.
329 Cf. Connolly, "Catechesis," in *New Life*, 87. According to the speculative description of the simple case technique by Tonti-Filippini, he indicates that

The Dignity of Human Procreation

is God who creates the soul of every human person that is brought into the world. God creates in every means chosen to transmit human life. However, the moral problem does not depend solely on whether God creates or not, instead, it comes from the means chosen by man to actualize his own role as one who pro-creates with God. As we have tried to indicate above, the transmission of life human life outside nature's designated context of conjugal love, corresponding to the nature of the person detracts from the dignity that is connatural to human procreation.

1.5. Summary

Drawing from the above articulations on both theological and anthropological bases, the rationale for situating or limiting the source of procreation to the conjugal act is the unity that encapsulates the corporal and spiritual nature of the couple and of the child to be born of that act. The anthropological and ontological structure of the conjugal act requires that there be no intentional separation in its unitive and procreative aspects. To arrive at the conclusion that the conjugal act is the only appropriate act upon which new life must ensue does not need to be shown dramatically, this is impossible. It is only by rigorous moral reasoning on the nature of man and of the goods of marriage that this conclusion is possible. The assertion that only the conjugal act is worthy of human life is based on the anthropology of the spouses and of the child to be generated inasmuch as they are human beings. It is equally derived from the divine law which informs us of creation being a specific act of love. God has made it to be so and man is not free to dismantle it. This explains why human procreation is deprived of its perfection when it is achieved without the conjugal act of the couple or realized outside the womb. The conjugal act is the expression or manner in which the man and woman as husband and wife respond to their mission of sharing in the mystery of personal communion and in the

---

the couple can engage in a sexual intercourse as a means of obtaining sperm to be used for IVF. This is carried out at the prescription of the medical personnel similar to what obtains in the GIFT method. The difference is that while in the GIFT fertilization occurs *in vivo*, in the simple case it occurs *in vitro*. What is important to note is that the sexual act, if it occurs, it is only for the sake of obtaining sperm in order to avoid masturbation condemned already.

creative work of God as Creator and Father. The sexual act of the couple is the act that reveals the apex of the couples' love for each other as a sharing in the life and love of the procreative act of God who creates out of love and in love. Being as it is, the conjugal act remains the source and the perfect environment suitable to express the point where God once again re-enacts his act of creation. The conjugal act therefore has a determined content of structure, purposes and intrinsic laws. It is by virtue of the nature of the conjugal act, corresponding to the totality of the person that the moral prohibition of the simple case IVF-ET is explained. That is, the unity of the human person in body and soul, makes it meaningful to maintain, that there is an intrinsic connection between the unitive and procreative aspects of the conjugal act. And so, the defenders of this principle agree that both dimensions of the sexual act are such that their meanings are dependent on each other. This is precisely why the simple case IVF procedure merits the negative judgment as a means of human procreation, a procedure that circumvents the conjugal act.

C. The Child Is Begotten, Not Made

1.1. An Overview of the Argument

We understand in the Catholic moral teaching that with the immense worth of human life as a being created in the image and likeness of God, a being that stands apart from other created beings by virtue of rationality and transcendence, the dignity of his origin corresponds to that of his nature. The generation of human life has its source in the conjugal act where God the Creator bequeaths to the couple the gift of life. God alone is the Originator and Giver of life, and he has established marriage as the natural environment suitable for the reception and nurturing of human life. Following this natural order of God's design, the child is not made but begotten. This implies that the couple that generate children by means of the conjugal act share their own nature with them and remain equal in dignity and right with them as human beings. In this manner, begetting a child indicates bringing into existence one's kind such that the young life and the old remain genetically the same but individually unique. But, to make a child by man gives the idea of bringing into existence a life that is alienated from its makers and suggests forcefully the power of domination over the new life. This concept of "making" does not convey the same meaning when used with reference to God because His activity is of a different level and kind from human actions. We can say: "God makes man" without any suspicion of manipulation, his own acting is perfect not like the actions of humans that are imperfect and deserve regulations.

In the teaching of the Instruction on human procreation, the Catholic Magisterium judges the simple case IVF to be morally illicit because it represents a procedure that "makes" a child rather than "begets" a child. While some theological opinions disagree with this conclusion, some uphold it and make efforts to show how true and reasonable the magisterial judgment is. The central arguments here from the point of view of theology and anthropology are the affirmations that: (1) human life is a gift of God to be begotten and not made; (2) the intrinsic and extrinsic dimensions of the simple case have a meaning of its own, a meaning that indicates domination over the young life; (3) a gift is not grabbed or forced but received and no one has a right to a gift, it depends on the giver to bestow his gift to whomever he chooses. It behoves on the receiver to respect the intention of the giver without abusing the gift or the means of its reception. In a word, the logic of the simple case IVF-ET is that of productivity and not procreativity.

1.2. The Child as a Gift of God in Marriage

That human life is a Gift of God does not appear to be a matter of controversy among Catholic theologians, at least in theory everyone seems accept this thesis. Catholic moral theologians opposed to the simple case technique of procreation emphasize or rather agree with *Donum Vitae* that a married couple has no right to a child, for a child is not an object to be possessed or owned in the manner of material things. A child is rather a gift of God, the supreme and most gratuitous gift of marriage.[330] The spouses have right

---

330 Cf. *Donum Vitae*, II, B/8: "A true and proper right to a child would be contrary to the child's dignity and nature. The child is not an object to which one has a right, nor can he be considered as an object of ownership: rather, a child is a gift, 'the supreme gift' and the most gratuitous gift of marriage, and is a living testimony of the mutual giving of his parents. For this reason, the child has the right, as already mentioned, to be the fruit of the specific act of the conjugal love of his parents; and he also has the right to be respected as a person from

only to perform those acts which are connatural with them and pertain to their marital union, acts which are ordered to the generation of children. In the Bible we read that God created mankind in his image and likeness (Gen. 1:27); and that the sons are a gift of God and the fruit of the womb, a reward (Psalm 127:3). John Paul II expresses this truth about human life when he says: "in God the life of the human being has its eternal source in a unique way, the human being whom he himself fashions in his own image when he quickens in the mother's womb."[331]

Since God is the Giver of life, it suggests that He is still directly involved in every act of procreation and the image of His involvement can be clearly felt when the generation of the child is brought about in marriage and through the specific action of the couple's sexual intercourse. The Instruction *Donum Vitae* affirms this truth when it stresses that the moral judgment about techniques of artificial procreation must not disregard the fact that the child is the fruit of the love union between the spouses.[332] That is why some theologians insist that the image or meaning of the child as a gift from God is absent in the simple case procedure. For instance, May argues that it is only through the conjugal act that human life is received and accepted as a gift from God. According to him, marriage is full of gifts and the gift of a child is still a symbol and fruit of the marital communion that is opened to the gift of new life. First, the husband and wife in marital communion are an expression of mutual self-gift of each other. It is only within this noble and holy context of self-giving and reception that the greater gift of a child is worthily received.

Furthermore, according to May, to underscore the relevance of the conjugal act as the appropriate act that brings out the meaning of human life

---

   the moment of his conception." See also Connolly, "Catechesis," in *The Gift of Life*, 86.
331 John Paul II, "Easter's Gift of Life," in *The Gift of Life*, 246.
332 Cf. *Donum Vitae*, II, A/1: "For human procreation has specific characteristics by virtue of the personal dignity of the parents and of the children: the procreation of a new person, whereby the man and the woman collaborate with the power of the Creator, must be the fruit and the sign of the mutual self-giving of the spouses, of their love and of their fidelity." The Instruction in this statement makes reference *Gaudium et Spes*, n. 50.

as a gift, it is necessary to distinguish between a marital act and a genital act. For him,

> The marital or conjugal act is not simply a genital act between a man and a woman who happen to be married. Husbands and wives have the capacity to engage in genital acts, as do nonmarried males and females, because of their sexual nature and their endowment with genitalia. But they have the capacity to (and the right) to engage in the marital act because they are spouses, i.e., husbands and wives.[333]

In the foregoing expressions, May tries to establish that human life is a special kind of gift from God reserved for those who have made themselves worthy for it by first donating and receiving themselves in conjugal union. It is not dependent on the capability of getting it either by technical means or by other dehumanizing means, but through a worthy and moral way befitting the personal dignity of the human person. A man and a woman who by their marital union make themselves responsible in their mutual love-giving and mutual reception of selves, equally make themselves worthy of sharing in the privilege of being co-creators with God. This implies that the total mutual giving and receiving of each other as husband and wife in a life-long commitment makes them worthy of being parents. It is on this basis that the teaching of the Church as repeated in *Donum Vitae* on the principle of inseparability of the two meanings of the conjugal act becomes evident and profound. May would insist;

> While husbands and wives have the right to engage in the marital act and, through it, to receive the gift of life, they do not have the right to a child. They do not have the right because a child, like them, a person, a being that is *sui iuris*. A child is not a thing which others can possess or own, nor is it an act to which persons can have rights.[334]

May's critique of the simple case procedure reveals his understanding that artificial fertilization is a form of "producing" or "making" human life but this obviously violates the goods of marriage and of the rights of the human person. Since human life is a gift from God, it is always wrong to employ ways of manipulating this life into being through technical efficiency. As a basic principle of *Donum Vitae* states, "what is technically possible is not

---

[333] May, "The Simple Case of In Vitro Fertilization and Embryo Transfer," 33.
[334] Ibid., 34.

for that very reason morally admissible,"³³⁵ it becomes apparent that the choice to procreate outside the marital act is an expression of counting more on the efficiency of the power of the technology than on seeking a means that respects human life at least in its origin.

By way of comparison, May in his argument likens the gift of life to the word that proceeds from God. Human life is designed by God to issue or proceed from the conjugal act like God's word proceeding from his mouth. The Divine word is precious and bears His imprints. That is how human life is felt when it proceeds from the conjugal act. May explains claims that,

> Human beings ought not to be made. They ought not to be made because they are human persons. And human persons I submit, are like 'words' that God speaks. Human persons are the beings made in the image and likeness of God (Gen. 1:28). As such they are his living icons, his words.... human beings God *created words*, ought, like the uncreated word who became and is one of them, to be 'begotten, not made.' They are begotten in the marital act; they are made in *in vitro* fertilization, homologous as well as heterologous.³³⁶

Thus, we have the impression that May believes that the most straightforward theological reason against the simple case IVF is that human life ought to be 'begotten, not made,' for in the conjugal act, the couple 'do' something to receive the blessing of marriage and not something they 'make.' May explains the difference between 'making' and 'doing' as follows:

> In 'making,' the action proceeds from an agent or agents to something produced in the external world. Autoworkers, for instance, produce cars; cooks produce meals; bakers produce cakes; etc. such action is transitive insofar as it passes from the acting subject(s) to an object fashioned by him or her (them). In this kind of human activity, governed by the rules of art, interest centers on the item made (and usually those which do not measure up to the standard are discarded – or at any rate, they are little appreciated). Those who produce the products made may be morally good autoworkers or cooks or bakers or they may be morally bad, but our interest in 'making' is the product, not the producers, and we would prefer to have good cars from morally wicked autoworkers than 'lemons' from morally good ones. In another mode of human activity – 'doing' – the action abides in the acting subject(s). The action is immanent and is governed by the requirement

---

335 *Donum Vitae*, Intro. 4.
336 William E. May, "*Donum Vitae*: Catholic Teaching concerning Homologous IVF," in *Philosophy and Medicine* 53, 3 (1997): 87. See similar argument from the same author in his *Catholic Bioethics and the Gift of Human Life*, 87.

of prudence, not by the rules of art. If the action is good, it perfects the agent(s); if bad, degrades and dehumanizes them.... When human life is given through the marital act, it comes, as we have seen, as a 'gift' crowning the act itself. The conjugal act is not an act of 'making.' It is not a transitive act issuing from the spouses and terminating in some object distinct from them. Rather, it is an act freely chosen by them to express their marital union, one open to the gift of life.[337]

Therefore, May's argument indicates that the simple case IVF changes the meaning of generating human life from being an immanent act of procreation to being a transitive act of "making" or "production." Rhonheimer seems to support May's opinion when he expresses that human life generated in the conjugal act is a doing and not a making or producing. For him, in the conjugal act, the couples give God a befitting space or favorable environment for a divine creative act to occur. In his words, "The conjugal act of the parents gives 'space' and occasion to this divine creative act; as such it is truly a 'service of life,' but not a dominion over life.' 'Service of life,' in relationships between human beings, can be understood – as opposed to 'dominion over life' – only as love,"[338] and this appears to be opposed by the choice to procreate outside the conjugal act in in vitro.

John Haas has also criticized artificial procreation arguing that human life is not to be 'made' but to be generated through an act of love of the couple. He shares the same views with other theologians who defend the magisterial teaching against the simple case from the perspective that children are begotten and not made by men. He notes,

> Human beings bear the image and likeness of God. They are to be reverenced as sacred. Never are they to be used as a means to an end, not even to satisfy the deepest wishes of an infertile couple. Husbands and wives "make love," they do not "make babies." They give expression to their love for one another, and a child may or may not be engendered by that act of love. The marital act is not a manufacturing process, and children are not products. Like the Son of God

---

337 May, "The Simple Case of In Vitro Fertilization," 35; Ibid., "Catholic Teaching Concerning Homologous IVF," 81–82. Aristotle and St. Thomas Aquinas have labored to make the distinction between these two significant words: "doing" and "making." For details, see Aristotle, *Metaphysics*, Bk. 9, c. 8, 1050a23–1050b1; St. Thomas Aquinas, *In IX Metaphysicorum*, lect. 8, n. 1865; *Summa Theologiae*, 1, 4, 2, ad 2; 1, 14, 5, ad 1; 1, 181, 1.
338 Rhonheimer, *Ethics of Procreation and the Defense of Human Life*, 166.

himself, we are the kind of beings who are "begotten, not made" and, therefore, of equal status and dignity with our parents.[339]

For Haas, in performing those acts proper to marital union with the openness, disposition and readiness to have a child, the couples are in such an attitude and action not of a making but of begetting the child. Through the power of God the Creator, the couple in their love-union, are empowered to bring forth the new life not strictly as the work of their hands but as the gift of God through their own marital act. Because the child is a gift of God received and nurtured in the context of marriage, the couple's role is that of cooperation with God to create a new life inherently and immensely of the same moral status as the humanity of his parents. In fact, as John Paul II talking about the rights of human beings, he indicates that "among the most important of these rights, mention must be made of the right to life, an integral part of which is the right of the child to develop in the mother's womb from the moment of conception."[340] This is to emphasize that the child is a gift, like every gift, he is not merited but gratuitously given by God in marriage.

1.3. An Instrumental Logic of Productivity Implied in the Technology

It is widely maintained by theological views opposed to the simple case IVF that this procedure carries with it the logic of productivity and not procreativity. For instance, in an article written by Ignaccio Carrasco de Paula,[341] he understands artificial fertilization to stand in sharp contrast and antagonistic to the dignity of human life. He observes that procreation suggests that human behavior sets the biological conditions necessary to enable a new human being to be conceived.[342] He feels that technology

---

339 John Haas, "Begotten Not Made: A Catholic View of Reproductive Technology," on https://www.usccb.org/issues-and-action/human-life-and-dignity/reproductive-technology/begotten-not-made-a-catholic-view-of-reproductive-technology. Accessed on 12 January 2015.
340 John Paul II, *Centessimus Annus*, 1 May 1991: in *AAS* 88 (1991): 851–852.
341 Ignaccio Carrasco de Paula, "Discerning Medically Assisted Procreation: Key Concepts of the Magisterium of the Catholic Church," in *Medicina e Morale* 5 (2013): 997–1007.
342 Ibid., 1001.

tends to build a child but marital act procreates a child. For him, artificial fertilization in general contains an inherent logic of production and reproduction of a material into identical copies. And so he observes,

> A person is neither a thing nor a simple copy representative of its species: each human individual is a unique being, inimitable and irreplaceable. Procreation follows a logic given to the person, such as the logic of benevolence [freely wanting good for another], the logic of the unconditional gift. Production and reproduction also have their logic, but is not the logic of benevolence; it is the logic of productivity, the logic of obtaining satisfactory results for those who put it into practice.[343]

Melina's opinion corroborates that of Carrasco de Paula when he submits that procreation outside the conjugal act is no procreation in the true sense but production. For him,

> The child is seen as a gift to be welcomed and not as a project to be built. Indeed, when the child is the result of a technical production and not a human action of self-giving, his condition of equal dignity with the parents and medical doctors is denied. As a 'product' he must meet the requests that commanded his planning. He forms part of a plan that tests and controls his quality.[344]

In this whole complication brought into play by the misuse of biomedical science and technology, Melina believes with many other theologians that parenthood becomes a myth when the technique employed does not assist the conjugal act but replaces it. For him the idea and value of parenthood is eclipsed in the simple case IVF. He feels that every form of IVF is suggestive of parenthood at any cost. But obviously, the logic of the simple case IVF is identical to artificial reproduction and inescapably leads to the myth of total parenthood by all cost; and this no longer respects either the personal dignity of the child or the leading role of the parents in their intimate love or the ultimate presence of God the Creator. Indeed, the feeling of God's presence at the beginnings of procreation is obscured in the replacement of the sexual act with technology. But, when the child is welcomed as a gift of God, it invokes an origin that is shared by the parents and children, that is constitutive of them both, and this is the basis of an authentic fatherhood

---

343 Ibid., 1002.
344 Melina, "The Intrinsic Logic of Interventions in the Field of Human Artificial Procreation: Ethical Aspects." 125.

or motherhood. While it is commonly acknowledged that in human family rightly founded by marital union of a man and woman, a love union that is open to new life, God is believed, felt and accepted as the Originator of the family and source of life. That is why Melina has argued that since IVF replaces the conjugal act, parents and children could incline to think that they are alienated from God in the whole event of procreation. This is persuasive because, when technology or the doctor comes to dominate and takes the place of the symbolic mediation of the spouses' bodies, the reality of God in their family is obscured and the image of human parenthood is deformed or deprived.

According to DeMarco, the biblical understanding of the human person is in terms of generation, a creative act of God where the imprint of God is communicated to man in such a way that man is made in the image and likeness of God. Procreation that is properly the cooperative responsibility of man with God retains this dignity when it proceeds from the conjugal act and by this expresses the gift of life as being begotten. But in artificial reproduction which the simple case IVF is considered in this light, is a mechanical model of human procreation which brings about "a twofold alienation: between the maker and the product, and between the maker and God."[345] He explains that:

> If a couple stands apart from their own offspring..., they are alienated from each other. Likewise, if a couple believes, as is consistent with the notion of 'reproduction,' that they are merely making or producing children [with the assistance of technology], then they do not believe they are cooperating in a way that intimately unites them with God. Thus, they are alienated from God.[346]

The consequence of this twofold alienation as DeMarco would want us to believe is that it leads man to lose his awareness of God, both as his own Creator and as the Creator of his children, as the one who sets his special seal of love on all human beings he creates. In furtherance, this alienation also causes a disconnection between love and power or as DeMarco would prefer "alienation of power from love." In fact, by separating power from

---

345 Donald T. DeMarco, "Catholic Moral Teaching and TOT/GIFT," in Donald McCarthy (ed.), *Reproductive Technologies, Marriage and the Church* (Braintree: The Pope John Centre, 1988), 139.
346 Ibid.

love in the order of reproduction, man loses sight of the God of love and seeks to become his own god, a god of power. The logic of artificial reproduction, therefore, can lead to atheism,[347] because it can appear to take the place of God or can diminish the active presence of God in human procreation. DeMarco's claim, one would think, needs to be understood in the context of technological arrogance of subjugating the origin of the child's life by technical efficiency.

Connolly reasons that this procedure "is in itself and objectively a process dominated by ideas of efficiency, usefulness, etc., independent of good intentions of future parents."[348] This idea was equally expressed at the presentation of the Instruction *Donum Vitae* by Ratzinger as the then President of the Congregation for the Doctrine of the Faith. According to him, the human being is always a "someone" and never a "something," always a "subject" and not an "object." He notes that the logic of some artificial procreative technologies *per se* constitutes "a relationship of inequality between the technician (who produces) and that which is produced, and therefore it is a relationship of dominion of the one over the other."[349] He equally argues that it is a misconception to think that the technique of artificial procreation does not possess any truth of its own but the human intention alone that gives ontological meaning to things. His view is rather in the contrary, noting that the technique of artificial procreation possesses the truth of a relationship of domination and inequality between the child, his parents and the technician.

Ratzinger further explains that the use of a technique to sunder the unitive and procreative dimensions of the conjugal act as a means of achieving a child, results not in procreation strictly speaking but in production. In other words, procreation implies a cooperation of spouses with God in the context of true conjugal act for the conception of new life. This new life must come as the fruit of the love union, an act and symbol of total self-donation and reception between the spouses. According to him,

> The conjugal act, in which are placed the conditions for the beginning of new life, does not create any relationship of 'production' between parents and children;

---

347 Ibid.
348 Connolly, "In Vitro Fertilization," in *New Life*, 61.
349 Cf. Liptak, *The Gift of Life*, 9.

by it the child is generated, not produced. The spouses place an act of love in the reciprocal gift of themselves and the child that can arise from this act is the gift of God's creative love. He or she is entrusted to the parents to be received by them with gratitude and infinite respect.[350]

It seems obvious, following theological opinions in support of the magisterial conclusion on the simple case IVF to conclude, that this procedure portrays the new life as an object to be possessed; and contains within it the impression of productivity subject to control and efficiency. This completely gives a meaning that is dehumanizing to the new life and represents an act of contradiction to the dignity of the Child and the couples.

1.4. The Child Is Not a Means of Fulfilling Parents' Desire

One of the arguments used by proponents of the simple case IVF-ET revolves around the need to fulfill the couple's desire of having children because a child is a good to marriage. Hence, the desire for a child is good and as such using the procedure as a last resort would be morally right. In other words, the use of this procedure for the generation of a child is good inasmuch as it fulfills the desire of the couple. The basic question from the opposing opinion has been if the child should be a means to an end, the end here being the fulfillment of the couple to be parents. It would imply that the couple's desire for the child is not for the good of the child but for the good of themselves. The child here becomes a means to their fulfillment, the joy of parenthood. In other words, the couple desire parenthood but the child is only a means to achieve this goal, this can be discerned from the technique of the simple case IVF and this is a common feature in all techniques of artificial procreation. This is not to suggest that the desire to be a parent in itself is wrong but that when this desire is expressed in a way that disregards the dignity of the child in its origin, it becomes clear that the desire is inordinate. Rhonheimer takes up this issue when he writes:

> ... IVF therefore makes the existence of others dependent on our desires and on our causal will, [...]. Just as the undesirability of a child does not justify killing it, so the desire for a child does not justify its production, that is, its being wanted

---

350 Ibid., 14.

causatively. In fact, in each of the cases the value of the concrete life is made dependent on the desires, on the will, and therefore on the power of others.[351]

The consequences of this according to Rhonheimer is that it becomes inevitable to say: you live because and in the measure in which we wanted it. We must accept human life because we want it and in the measure in which it is wanted; it cannot be that human life exists only because and in the measure, in which it is accepted, desired, or willed. We would certainly not accept that attitude towards ourselves, neither can we relate to others in this manner.[352] In his view, it is wrong to generate human life simply because it is desired, a mere desire is not sufficient to have a child, the means for realizing this desire must be licit, otherwise this would be contrary to the dignity of the child to be generated. Hence, with particular reference to the case under consideration, the dissolution of the link between the unitive and the procreative meanings by means of a technique of production is against the nature of human procreation. This is so "not because it violates the fact of nature, but because it contradicts the unconditional acceptance of a human life, and because precisely this kind of unconditional acceptance is 'according to nature' for man."[353] In this sense, Rhonheimer indicates that the generation of human life outside the conjugal act based on the will of the couple or simply to fulfill their desire implies a production of an object rather than a consequence of a doing (*praxis*) of the conjugal act from which life is created. Therefore, in this case the will could be described as the 'instrumentalization of the generation of a human being so as to fulfil the desire for a child.'[354]

---

351 Rhonheimer, *Ethics of Procreation and the Defense of Human Life*, 170.
352 Ibid.
353 Ibid. The author would like us to believe that in the light of practical reason, the generation of human life outside the conjugal act and as a product of causative will contradicts the golden rule, the most fundamental principle of justice for all humans. And so, it is an unjust act to subject the origin of human life to this condition of mere desire.
354 Ibid., 166. It is his conviction that the choice of conceiving a child in a test tube contains within itself a contradiction. In other words, the child as a good which the couple desire is given the image of an object because of the means chosen to realize this desire. "The presupposition of the argument in favour IVF is in effect that the desire for a child is a good. Why, on the whole, is it good to desire a child? Certainly not because it is a good to have desires, and

Germain Grisez joins the argument when he observes that fertility is a gift of God, who owes nothing to anyone. The children are part of the fulfillment of married life, a good of the marriage but not solely of the spouses but as a good in itself.[355] He believes that because of the value couples have for children, many couples especially those having infertility problem usually become so desperate that they seek medical assistance at any cost. But Grisez feels that it is morally right for couples with infertility challenge to seek medical help to overcome their condition but he thinks it is hard to see any good reason going to the great lengths that some do. He questions their agitation by saying that:

> That fixation is morally questionable. The emotional focus is on having the prospective baby as a concrete state of affairs – a goal, a desired object. Volitionally, a baby maybe sought to satisfy the intense emotional desire and to fulfill the married couple precisely insofar as that fulfillment is their own good. If so, the baby is not willed for his or her own sake, but as an instrumental good. This motivation is different from the normal case of a couple uprightly choosing to marry and have a family. They too, of course, can experience a strong desire to have a

---

the generation of a child fulfills those desires! The good is not in the first place in the fulfillment of the desire, rather in the obtainment of that which was the object of the desire. In the same way, the good of joy does not consist primarily in rejoicing, but in that which one rejoices; and the good of pleasure is not in the pleasure itself, rather it is in the object of this experience, in what is enjoyed. But why is it good to have a child? Certainly, because a child is a good. But why is it a good? If one does not wish to degrade the child to a simple means of fulfilling the desires of other people, he can only say: it is good precisely because the existence of a person in a way absolutely independently of every desire is already *per se* a good, and according to the requirement of justice [the 'golden rule'], it only can be desired as such a good. It is precisely this, however, which is negated with IVF, because it implies the acknowledgement of the birth of a new life as a 'good' precisely in the measure in which is an object of my causative will. Procreative technology is therefore a mode of action by which the person as the subject of action obscures, and even destroys, at least tendentially, the basis of his own freedom of self – determination to the good in general and to the just in particular. For this reason also, the separation of procreation and sexual union is not in conformity with man's nature, and precisely because it is opposed to reason, just as in order to gather wood, it is contrary to reason to saw off a branch on which one is sitting." Ibid., 174.

355 Germain Grisez, *The Way of the Lord Jesus, Vol. 3: Difficult Moral Questions* (Quincy: Franciscan Press, 1997), 246.

baby. But for such couple, having and raising children are included in the benefits of marital fulfillment, and they hope for this whole, complex good of marriage as an end. Thus, the couple need not and usually do not seek a prospective child precisely as a goal instrumental to an ulterior benefit for themselves.[356]

Although, Grisez observes that some technical means are used not to produce a child but to assist the conjugal act by removing the obstacles to its fruitfulness, in the same way it happens in other medical techniques to help in other bodily functions when abnormal conditions interfere with them. Therefore, the moral assessment of the legitimacy of the reproductive technique should consider both the intrinsic character of what is done and the motives for doing it. In this way he identifies two criteria: the character of the means and the motives for the action. He is also considering here the fact that some married couples desire the child not for the child's sake as a good in itself but for their selfish fulfillment. Thus, "using technical means to assist the marital act's natural fruitfulness is morally acceptable, but doing so to satisfy desire for a prospective child as a means to parental fulfillment vitiates any use of technical means."[357] But he also feels that even if the child is desired for this reason and the morally acceptable technique is employed, the whole action will be morally wrong because of the intention of the couple for using such a means. He thinks that those who are not trying to produce a baby by technical means but are only using technique to assist marital intercourse, and even those who are engaging only in unassisted intercourse, may nevertheless be acting with the unsound motivation of wanting a child for their self-fulfillment. It is Grisez's submission that:

> All married couples who desire a child should examine their motives and criticize them, to ensure that they are not interested in the baby as one among many things they consider necessary or helpful for their self-fulfillment. They should hope for a baby as a gift who, while making their love fruitful, will be loved for his or her own sake. Having intercourse with that hope in mind is not using the marital act as a means of producing a child.[358]

Actually, Grisez's contention captures succinctly the sentiment of the Vatican's Instruction. The Latin name for the document *Donum Vitae*

---

356 Ibid, 246–247.
357 Ibid, 245.
358 Ibid, 248–249.

translates as "gift of life." It is precisely with this understanding that he argues and of which his appeal to the intention or motivation of the couple alongside the means employed becomes very significant. He gives the impression that the intention of the couples and the means of achieving procreation could make it morally right or wrong. If both or either of them is wrong, the act will certainly be morally illicit.

Kathleen Curran Sweeney observes that although the desire for a child in marriage is strong and understandable but it cannot justify the use of any means to achieve such a desire. She affirms the teaching of the Magisterium that couples do not have a right to a child rather it is the child who has intrinsic right to be born in marriage and strictly through the conjugal act. She notes,

> A couple who takes the position that they will do anything to have a child, expresses a willfulness and possessiveness over the child's existence. A married couple cannot say they have a right to a child. A child is not a piece of property to be possessed by the parents. A child is a human person of equal dignity to the parents and cannot be considered as an object to be desired and possessed. Rather, a couple needs to see the child as a gift and welcome him as a blessing, the fruit of the love they offer each other in the conjugal act. The conjugal act expresses the nuptial meaning of the sexual body, the self-gift of husband and wife to each other.[359]

In fact, the good intentions of couples to have a child through IVF-ET are not sufficient moral requirements to make their actions morally right. The meaning implied in this technique of human fertilization is one of possession which destroys the good intention or rather contradicts the good intention the couple might have besides the good intention of the medical personnel willing to help. The position of *Dignitas Personae* gives us the basis to make some conclusions on the subject under consideration:

> Certainly, techniques aimed at removing obstacles to natural fertilization, as for example, hormonal treatments for infertility, surgery for endometriosis, unblocking of fallopian tubes or their surgical repair, are licit. All these techniques may be considered *authentic treatments* because, once the problem causing the infertility has been resolved, the married couple is able to engage in conjugal

---

[359] Kathleen Curran Sweeney, "The Technical Child: In Vitro Fertilization and the Personal Subject," at http://www.christendom-awake.org/pages/may/sweeney.htm. Accessed on 19 January 2015.

acts resulting in procreation, without the physician's action directly interfering in that act itself. None of these treatments replaces the conjugal act, which alone is worthy of truly responsible procreation.[360]

1.5. Summary

This section has explored certain opinions that the simple case IVF-ET bespeaks the language of making contrary to begetting. Since this is morally wrong, relevant theological arguments are presented in support of the thesis that human life is begotten not made. First, it is argued that human life is a gift of God in marriage, a gift that is only received through the conjugal act. Proponents of this theological view, insist that when human conception occurs outside the conjugal act, or rather when the child is not the fruit of the specific conjugal act of the couple but the result of some scientific manipulations, the child is being produced or made and not begotten or procreated. In this perspective, the sense of life being a gift from God is lost or obscured.

Furthermore, we have indicated that defenders of the magisterial stance have claimed that human life cannot be a means to an end in the manner of being produced for the sake of fulfilling the yearning of couples who desire to achieve parenthood. This is not to say, the desire for parenthood is wrong in itself but that desiring the child not for the child's good but for the sake of fulfilling some desires of the parents is morally illicit. When the child comes as a result of the causative will of the parents in which case everything is done to have him through technological efficiency, as it is the case in the simple case IVF, it becomes an act of injustice against the child's dignity. The child has equal inviolable right as those of his parents or the doctor as a human person and so cannot be desired merely for their fulfillment as if he were an object for possession and not a human being. These factors constitute some of the moral problems of the simple case IVF-ET and that is why it cannot be considered a morally licit means of generating human life.

---

360 *Dignitas Personae*, n. 13.

Synthesis of the Chapter

The magisterial stance on the simple case IVF-ET as articulated in the recent Instructions *Donum Vitae* and *Dignitas Personae*, has got remarkable affirmation and defense from some renowned moral theologians as illustrated in the foregoing discussion. No doubt, these moral theologians argue from various perspectives but they have some converging views central to the advancement of the Church's rejection of the simple case IVF-ET. They take into consideration the anthropological and theological perspectives of man in his historical and redemptive experiences, in order to affirm that the simple case IVF-ET is a morally illicit means of procreation. For them, the simple case IVF procedure cannot be considered truly as an assisted technique of procreation because the conjugal act cannot be delegated to another person as implied in this procedure. In the light of this, the procedure is offensive and contrary to the dignity of human procreation and in another sense, marriage as a theological environment where God re-creates human life is brought into disrepute. Indeed, the intrinsic nature of this procedure conveys the language of production and not procreation, and so the child to be conceived is likely subjected to the category of "something" and not "someone."

The principle of inseparability which based on the substantial unity of the person, affirms that the unitive and the procreative meanings of the conjugal act must not be sundered or dissolved by human initiative, constitutes the basis upon which this procedure is judged unacceptable. In the light of this teaching, the simple case IVF-ET in which human conception cannot be attributed to the specific act of the conjugal sexual act, is not a worthy method for human procreation. Furthermore, the theologians we have studied insist that human life is a gift of God to be begotten in the context of the conjugal act and not made through the manipulation of technology. As a gift, no one claims the right to children. Couples only have rights to perform those legitimate acts of love that pertain to marriage but do not have the right to or can claim ownership of life. Gifts even in the ordinary sense cannot be grabbed by force, otherwise the act of receiving the gift would change its meaning in the negative. This is precisely the impression the simple case IVF-ET like other means of artificial procreation that occur outside the conjugal act represents. It would be an act of injustice to subject human life to quality control and also to seek a child as a means of fulfilling the parent's desire for parenthood.

This theological position understands, however, that a medically assisted procreation is an intervention in the generation of human life that respects and maintains the unity of the love union and procreative dimensions of the conjugal act, it also preserves the dignity of the person by not replacing the conjugal act or subjecting human conception to technological determination outside the maternal body. It has been indicated that the simple case IVF rather than seeks to heal the pathology of infertility, seeks to address human desires instead. On the whole, opposed views insist that procreation outside the sphere of the maternal body degrades the dignity of children, marriage and procreation. Undoubtedly, the problem of human infertility is staring us in the face but to intervene with the simple case IVF-ET procedure would not seem to be a better option on moral grounds. In the light of this difficulty, what suggestions or proposals could be offered as a contribution to the debate called for by the Magisterium by means of the Instruction *Donum Vitae*?

General Evaluation and Conclusion

The debate on the morality of the simple case IVF-ET within the Catholic circle has been interesting and complex. This debate is interesting because it can contribute towards broader and perhaps clearer perspectives on the question of intervention in human procreation in the emerging horizons in biomedicine. It is complex because it requires a comprehensive vision of the human person, an adequate evaluation of the nature of this technology as a human act and the appreciation of the pains of infertility for married persons. From the time of the publication of the Instruction *Donum Vitae* in 1987 to the present time, the debate has been characterized principally as an interaction between those who seem to justify exceptions to some moral rules on the grounds of proportionalistic method of moral reasoning and those who hold that there are some moral norms that must be acknowledged to be absolute, norms that pertain to the so-called intrinsically evil acts by virtue of their moral object. In the foregoing, we have presented a review of the magisterial teachings of the Catholic Church on artificial procreation from the teachings of Pius XI, Pius XII and Paul VI. The Instruction *Donum Vitae* reveals an anthropology that is in a deep continuity and consistency with the previous teachings of the Magisterium. We have also tried to articulate the arguments of the dissenting theological opinions on the simple case with the critiques of the Instruction's consultation claims, logic, derivation and application of moral norms on methods of human procreation. The defending opinions of Catholic theologians who accept the arguments and conclusions of the Instruction on the simple case have also been presented as a response to the dissenting views and as a way of deepening *Donum Vitae*'s judgment.

At this point let us quickly recall that the Instruction *Donum Vitae* defines the simple case as a homologous IVF and ET procedure that is free of any compromise with the abortive practice of destroying embryos and with masturbation.[361] This mode of generating human life appears to the dissenting theologians primarily as a positive, life-giving technology serving

---

361 *Donum Vitae*, II, B/5.

a perfectly legitimate human desire to have children. As we noted in Chapter Two, inasmuch as the opinion of the dissenting theologians may be valid in its own dimension in respect of the fact that the child is one of the goods of marriage, there are certain aspects that remain problematic if considered in the light of the natural law and the Catholic moral teachings on the nature of the person and on the dignity of human procreation. Inspired by previous magisterial teachings of the Church as presented in Chapter One of this work, the Instruction *Donum Vitae* asserts that the simple case procedure may not be characterized by all that ethical negativity found in extracorporeal fertilization, however, considering the goods of marriage and the dignity of the person, this means of generating human life is objectively disordered. Therefore, in the following section, we will attempt to present briefly the results or insights gained from the research.

1. The Context of the Research

Our study is contextual and limited to the moral and theological perspectives on the simple case and has its objectives to stimulate interest, offer interpretations and clarifications regarding the debate on this mode of human fertilization. This discussion, attempts to respond to the invitation for dialogue by the Magisterium on the new challenges in artificial procreation. No doubt, the Magisterium has ruled out on the acceptability of the simple case because it judges it to be an immoral mode of generating human life, but a continuous debate on this question would not be unnecessary or superfluous. This study offers us the opportunity to be better informed of what Catholic theologians are saying about the subject we are dealing with. This can give us the basis of deepening our awareness of the history and principles that guide the Church's moral judgment on this procedure as well as contemporary interpretations and applications of these principles with respect to the new reproductive technologies. In fact, the opinions of moral theologians blessed with the requisite experience and capacity are invaluable, because they attempt to clarify the principles of the document since they are not self-evident and more so, that the Instruction is intended to be a moral guide but not a theological treatise. And more importantly, for the fact that the discordance of views among Catholic theologians and pastors on this matter, it is possible that it can constitute a problem for the less informed couples and perhaps sets them in a state of dilemma in their search for a pastoral guide on the problem of infertility/childlessness. From the literature available to us for this research, the so-called simple case IVF-ET is presented as a hypothetic procedure, a theoretical problem. To this extent, our presentation of the problem is theoretically based without actual clinical indications except in the aspects that are similar to standard homologous IVF-ET. We have the impression that many authors who contribute in this debate on the simple case actually do not make a clear distinction between the simple case and the standard homologous IVF-ET. While the former is still on the level of a possibility, the latter has been in practice from the first successful case of IVF-ET since 1978.

2. The Status of the Simple Case IVF-ET

First, the simple case is not yet realistic but it is proposed as a possibility. From *Donum Vitae*'s descriptive definition of this procedure as well as other theological views and protocols, this procedure would practically not be feasible given the present practice of IVF-ET. The analysis of the situation by Tonti-Filippini is particularly instructive and insightful regarding this procedure. According to him, the assessment of this simple case reveals that it would not be a practical procedure. The reason is that the current state of the art of the standard IVF-ET has given doubts that the simple case could be performed considering the moral issues and risks associated with it. That is, the risks and burden of the procedure would be too enormous for it to be performed to get desired results. It is likely too that the physicians might be unwilling to follow all the ethical rigors of this procedure that gives an indication of a very minimal rate of success, a situation that possibly makes both the physicians and couples to consider it disproportionately burdensome.[362] The simple case IVF-ET is far from being "simple" to be achieved because it is ethically complex besides other problematic aspects.

---

362 Cf. Tonti-Filippini, "IVF: The Role of the Physician," 71.

3. Some Basic Points of Agreement between the Pros and Cons on the Simple Case

There are several aspects that the pros and cons arguments on the simple case find agreement. The first point is on marriage and the vocation of married couples to procreate. Both groups agree that marriage is the morally and naturally designed context for procreation and nurturing of children. They agree that the child conceived must be the fruit of his parent's love. Second, both opinions maintain a negative judgment on the heterologous IVF-ET. However, while the dissenting opinion, in so doing appeals to social reasons such as a discordant family identity problem, other theologians go deeper anthropologically into the problem of inseparability of the conjugal act. Third, all Catholic theologians agree following the Instruction's judgment, that human acts like masturbation, abortive practices and eugenics are morally wrong means to achieve human procreation. Fourth, Catholic theologians accept the Instruction's teaching on the inviolability of human life and the sanctity of the means of transmitting human life. Fifth, there is unity of opinions that medical technology is not contrary to the nature of man in terms of being used correctly to assist human procreation in certain circumstances of infertility. In other words, technology is a value and a gift of God in the service of man.

4. The Debate on the Simple Case Prior to *Donum Vitae*

From our presentation of the magisterial teachings relating to human procreation prior to *Donum Vitae*, the generation of human life outside the conjugal act is rejected by Pius XII based on the natural law teaching and the vision of the Church about marriage and procreation. The Pope seems to base his rejection of artificial insemination by husband as well as IVF-ET on four goods:

1. The dignity of husband and wife as the image of God.
2. Their fidelity to God and each other expressed in their bodily and spiritual union requires the exclusion of any action that contradicts the truth that conception be the direct fruit of their self-giving and acceptance.
3. Their responsibility or vocation to be co-creators with God that requires them to have a child in response to the language of their bodies. The

communion of love and life of the spouses is a sanctuary by which the Creator continues to create new human life, it is a mission entrusted to them.
4. Their obligation to accept the will of God or to fulfill the will of Providence to be biological parents or otherwise.

In view of these goods, the Pope judges that only the medical means that do not separate procreation from the conjugal act may be morally acceptable to assist infertile couples to have children.

In this period, theological discussions strictly on the simple case were merely evolving from the general debate on artificial insemination and IVF-ET. The dissenting theologians made allusions to the possibility of modifying the standard IVF-ET procedure to exclude deliberate destruction of human embryos, cryopreservation, gamete donation, masturbation and similar practices paving way to the so-called "the simple case IVF-ET." In such a context, they argue that the procedure would simply and properly meet the moral requirement of respecting the dignity of the person and could be used as medical assistance to the marital relationship to achieve procreation. Generally and basically, the two aspects of the argument are: the life of the child to be born and the nature of the conjugal act. Following Pius XII's teaching that did not condemn in principle interventions in human procreation, there were controversies among theologians on what constitutes the requirement for accepting as licit a particular method. This situation also contributed to the proposal by some scholars that the simple case could meet the criteria for acceptability.

5. The Debate after *Donum Vitae*

Sequel to the publication of *Donum Vitae*, theological discussions relating directly or indirectly to the simple case started receiving improved attention among Catholic and non-Catholic theologians. The Instruction directly proscribes the simple case giving the reason that it lacks the perfection connatural with the dignity of human procreation. With this straightforward rejection of the simple case, the dissenting theologians or as Sgreccia prefers to call them, "Possibilists," have continued to express optimism that this procedure could be achieved as a morally good means of assisting infertile couples to have children of their marriage. Talking about the debate on the simple case after *Donum Vitae* one can hardly do so without mentioning that the document has become central to any discussion on this procedure. While many authors have expressed deep appreciation and support for the Instruction, the dissenting theologians have attacked the document on claims pertaining to its methodology, argumentation, assumptions and consultation process much more than dwelling on the validity and relevance of the Instruction. In fact, substantially, the debate on the simple case before and after *Donum Vitae* largely revolves around the same concerns of respect for human life and the nature of the conjugal act. The Instruction as well as its defending argument essentially has to do with the justification of why procreation must be tied to the specific sexual act of the couple's love and not on the totality of marriage.

6. The Divergent Anthropologies and Approaches to the Simple Case

Generally, in this research, we have noticed that from purely anthropological and theological considerations, the two contrasting views in the debate have dissimilar visions and approaches to the simple case based on their particular understandings of the nature of the person, marriage and procreation. Although each group claims to have an adequate and personalist vision of the person, yet their views are seemingly irreconcilable with each other. For example, the Magisterium as well as its defending theologians on the transmission of human life, understands procreation to be a continuum that begins with the conjugal act, a personal act that cannot be replaced if procreation is to retain its intrinsic dignity. This view considers as a moral requirement the natural union of the couple's gametes in the context of marital act or at least a medical aid for it to unite within the body. But, the dissenting opinion in supporting the simple case procedure, seems to understand the nature of human procreation to consist in the union of the couple's gametes (even by artificial means), for this reason the bodily union of the spouses in conjugal act which allows the natural unity of their gametes to occur is not given a moral priority by these dissenting theologians. From another perspective, the dissenting theologians, although not all of them would accept, their position suggests that they see the body as an instrument of the person. And so, the couple's are merely means of getting gametes for the generation of life. Contrary to this, theologians opposed to the simple case, inspired by the Church's teaching see the person as a "unified totality" where the body is an expression of the person and not merely instrumental. This substantial unity of the person forms the basis for the moral judgment of the Magisterium on the transmission of human life.

7. The Conjugal Act as the Most Fundamental Principle for the Rejection of the Simple Case

In the course of this work we have observed that the central principle upon which depends the moral acceptability or otherwise of the simple case IVF-ET is the inseparability principle of the link between the two meanings of the conjugal act. The conjugal act is therefore a fundamental key that defines the generation of human life as an act of pro-creating with God and which retains and respects the dignity that is intrinsic to the person. This is the fundamental key that is absent in the simple case. The human person lives and exists in the material world as a composite of body and soul. The human body is a fundamental component of the person and manifests or expresses the person. The substantial unity of the person as body and soul accounts for the indissoluble connection between love union and procreation as well as allows for the expression of personal union through bodily union in the conjugal act. Essentially, this is the anthropological understanding that explains away the reason why the simple case that undermines this truth of human nature lacks the moral requirement of an authentic medical assisted procreation which *Donum Vitae* judges to be licit and recommends for infertile couples. However, the dissenting theological view maintains that an imperfect act is not by that very fact a moral wrong to reject the simple case that would bring remedy to the childless couples.

8. Other Principles against the Simple Case

Beyond the principle of inseparability there are other principles complementing this central principle, because the severance of the conjugal act from procreation has other consequences that pertain to those human values to be protected by these principles. These principles are: inviolability of human life, the child as a gift, human life as an end in itself and not a means to satisfy the quest for parenthood and that there is no intrinsic right to a child. All these are connected to the basic moral doctrine that the child is begotten and not made. That is, as a moral requirement the child is received in the conjugal act as a gift of God and not made as a product of technical actions in the laboratory. This is related to the moral law of natural justice that human life cannot be treated, either in its coming into being or in its existence, as a property to be owned but as a life to be nurtured with responsibility. The simple case IVF-ET is believed to speak the logic of ownership of the child that is contrary to the logic of human life as an end in itself. While the Church's teaching does not reject or foreclose in principle technology *per se* in human procreation, the simple case is rejected because it is considered to constitute a replacement to the conjugal act and not an aid to it.

9. Intentionality Is Not Sufficient in Itself to Justify the Use of the Simple Case

From our study it is obvious that the argument on the morality of the simple case IVF-ET is complex; it requires an adequate understanding of the object of this procedure as the primary and decisive element for a moral judgment. For advocates of the simple case, the object of this procedure cannot be derived exclusively from the object of the technique apart from the intention of the couple and their circumstances. In their view, the claim that the simple case is intrinsically evil cannot be taken for a good moral judgment to reject the simple case. Instead, they argue, the simple case IVF-ET can be morally licit insofar as it promotes the marital relationship as well as grants the fulfillment of the couple with children in their marriage. This theological opinion proposes that the moral evaluation of the simple case should take into consideration all the elements of the act: its object, circumstances and end, in order to make a conclusion based on its result. The theological position justifying the simple case IVF procedure portrays the dissenting theologians as promoters of the theological school of proportionalism or consequentialism. In their view, the resort to the simple case is only a requirement to overcome and complement what nature lacks, such that even without the conjugal act and the seemingly intrusive nature of the procedure, the good of having a child can compensate for any defect in it.

In the contrary, theologians who defend the judgment of the Instruction argued, that the good intention of the couple is not sufficient to justify the use of the simple case that has an inherently disordered moral object, because *embodiment* of the spouses that pertains to the basic criterion of procreation is missing. Besides, based on natural justice, human life cannot be used as a means to fulfill the desire to attain parenthood. Spouses do not have right to a child, if it were, the child would be less human and inferior to the life of his parents. It is therefore contrary to natural justice, the divine law and the dignity of the child to make good intention the principal determining condition for the morality or justification of the simple case IVF-ET. In consonance with the Catholic moral doctrine, the object of the human act (*finis operis*) as different from the intention of the actor (*finis operantis*) constitutes the determining factor of the evilness or goodness of an act, and this moral object is neither purely spiritual nor physical but an embodiment, a choice of action that occurs in a real world. To the extent that the intention of the spouses (*finis operantis*) is also significant in the overall judgment of the procedure alongside the circumstances, it cannot by itself render the procedure morally acceptable.

10. The Simple Case Offends against the Dignity of Human Procreation

For the fact that the simple case could be achieved without respect to the integrity of bodily union in a conjugal act makes it harmful and offensive to the dignity of human procreation. We can imply that inasmuch as this procedure deviates from the unity of the conjugal act and achieves fertilization of human life outside the body in a condition that subjects the child's origins to technical decisions of experts in the manner of producing objects, it cannot be judged morally worthy of human procreation. Hence, in this opinion, the simple case IVF-ET falls short of the moral requirement consistent with the dignity and right of the child to be the fruit of the specific act of conjugal love. The choice of the simple case as a means of procreation depicts contempt to the dignity of procreation in two ways. First, it attacks the dignity of the child by the presence of the "third party" in an act that requires the exclusivity of two-in-one intimacy, which is the source of the child as its fruit. Second, it makes the couple look irresponsible and abusive by allowing themselves to be used as simple objects or means in a procedure that disregards or destroys the dignity of the child in his origins. Consequently, the acceptability of the simple case should not depend on technical efficiency simply because it might result in a healthy child or avoid deliberate abortion and other harmful practices but in the nature that defines the procedure itself, namely, an act of "making" a child. In other words, the simple case "makes" a child while conjugal act begets a child, and human life is begotten not made, therefore, the simple case IVF-ET is a wrong mode of generating human life.

But, the question might be asked if human life can really come into existence if it were not first created or willed by God? In other words, if God makes it possible for life to be generated even in the unfamiliar way through the simple case IVF-ET, would it not imply that there are no strict or specified means of generating life except the concern about how that life should be nurtured? If the response is in the affirmative, then the marital relationship would be an uncompromising context for the transmission of human life but the specificity of the sexual act would only be an option. No doubt, this position has the possibility of posing other problematic situations but might not be morally or theologically based. This means that from the perspectives of morality and theology, it would be difficult to prove that the simple case IVF-ET contradicts any theological or moral rule since God has empowered man to subdue nature to his advantage. This line of reasoning is apparently erroneous and is obviously inferred from the arguments in support of the simple case. Indeed, the response to the above argument has been offered in the teaching of the Magisterium by showing what it means to attribute intrinsic evil to the simple case IVF-ET. A human act is evil or wrong due to a deprivation of moral goodness. This moral goodness or its absence, in any act, is determined by the eternal moral law, by the law of justice inherent in the very nature of God. The eternal moral law is the law of love: the love of God above all else and the love of neighbor as self. So an act is evil or wrong when it has a deprivation of the properly ordered love of God, neighbor, self. Any act contrary to that love is a wrong act. From our presentation of the teaching of the Instruction and the theological opinions which uphold and defend *Donum Vitae*'s position, the simple case IVF-ET for the fact that it deprives procreation of the conjugal act and equally subjects the new human life to a condition of both spiritual and physical harm, injustice and depreciation of moral worth, it is inherently contrary to true love and to human life. By this view, it is contrary to the eternal moral law and therefore morally wrong. There is no doubt that relying only on the law of nature the generation of human life can come about by any means inasmuch as the required natural condition of the sperm and egg are met for fertilization to occur. But, human procreation as we hinted previously, is not simply achieved by the external union of the gametes but about the union of persons in the exercise of married love. With this, it would not be reproduction because it is achieved following not just the law of nature but the natural law that guides all rational beings. It is this natural law and the eternal moral law, which inform man on the manner human generation should be achieved. Hence, the evaluation of the simple case IVF-ET as a morally wrong act is dependent not on the law of nature but on the natural moral law.

Finally, the justification of the simple case as a licit means of procreation by some Catholic moral theologians led by McCormick is an error in their understanding of the true nature of the human person and the moral requirement that the child should be the fruit of the specific act of conjugal love. It cannot be denied that the Instruction *Donum Vitae* has set a standard of moral judgment on medical interventions in human procreation and specifically judged as morally wrong the use of the simple case for the generation of human life. But, the Church's position does not appear abundantly evident to those who dissent and argue in favor of the simple case. Unfortunately, the dissenting theologians have not proved beyond every reasonable doubt that they are not in error just as their propositions are in most cases unpersuasive and ambiguous. Our study has its limitations as well because it cannot resolve all the issues at stake or pretend to have understood everything about this subject. Rather, one fact remains doubtless, it has made a contribution at least to provoke or motivate further investigations into the subject we have treated in this project. In fact, having attempted to present arguments of the pro and con theological groups on the simple case, it must be acknowledged that the discussion to prove convincingly why the simple case is licit or otherwise is not an easy task. Catholic moral theologians have enormous responsibility in this regard. During these years following the publication of *Donum Vitae* and its condemnation of the simple case IVF-ET, specific and clear discussions on this matter are scarce and still developing. We hope that precise and intensive interactions on the moral problems of this technique would grow as a contribution to *Donum Vitae*'s invitation to moral theologians for dialogue on the current challenges posed by new reproductive technologies. In addition to *Donum Vitae* and *Dignitas Personae*, the encyclicals *Veritatis Splendor* and *Evangelium Vitae* of John Paul II as well as publications of the Pontifical Academy for Life and other interventions of the Magisterium, can afford one with clear indications about both the approach and content of the evaluation of the problem we have tried to treat. Without doubts, the contributions of moral theologians both those who dissent and those who agree with the conclusion of the Magisterium as expressed in our study, altogether represents an investigation into the reality of this complex problem in the light of the Catholic faith. We can draw our conclusion with a statement from *Dignitas Personae*:

> Certainly, techniques aimed at removing obstacles to natural fertilization, as for example, hormonal treatments for infertility, surgery for endometriosis, unblocking of fallopian tubes or their surgical repair, are licit. All these techniques may be considered *authentic treatments* because, once the problem causing the infertility has been resolved, the married couple is able to engage in conjugal acts resulting in procreation, without the physician's action directly interfering in that act itself. None of these treatments replaces the conjugal act, which alone is worthy of truly responsible procreation.[363]

Since the simple case may not be considered as an authentic treatment for infertility because it replaces the specific personal act of conjugal love and does not permit procreation to be the result of conjugal act; and for the fact that it is not morally obliging to take extraordinary means involving avoidable great risks to both the life of the child to be born and the marital life of couples, the decision for adoption appears to be more reasonable for infertile couples than the choice of the simple case IVF-ET. Besides, the Catholic Magisterium has given some indications that infertile couples could legitimately utilize certain methods of homologous assisted insemination provided such techniques do not substitute for the conjugal act.

---

363 *Dignitas Personae*, n. 13.

Bibliography

Magisterium and other Statements from the Holy See

BENEDICT XVI, *Address to the Participants in the Symposium on the theme: "Stem Cell: What Future for Therapy?"* Vatican City, 16 September 2006. Found on http://academiavita.org/documents.php.

———, *Address to the Participants to the International Congress on: "The Christian Conscience in Support of Human Life,"* Vatican City, 24 February 2007. Found on http://academiavita.org/documents.php.

CONGREGATION FOR THE DOCTRINE OF THE FAITH, *Instruction on Respect for Human Life in Its Origin and On the Dignity of Human Procreation, Donum Vitae*, 22 February 1987: *AAS* 80 (1988): 70–102.

———, *Instruction Dignitas Personae on Certain Bioethical Questions and the Dignity of the Person*, 20 June 2008: *AAS* 100 (2008): 858–887.

JOHN PAUL II, Encyclical *Centesimus Annus*, 1 May 1991, in AAS 83 (1991): 793–867.

———, Encyclical *Veritatis Splendor*, 6 August 1993: *AAS* 85 (1993): 1133–1169.

———, Encyclical *Evangelium Vitae*, 25 March 1995: *AAS* 87 (1995): 401–522.

———, *Address on the Occasion of the 10th Anniversary of the Foundation of the Pontifical Academy for Life* (Vatican City, February 20–22, 2004), in Juan De Dios Vial Correa and Elio, Sgreccia (eds.), *The Dignity of Human Procreation and Reproductive Technologies: Anthropological and Ethical Aspects*, Libreria Editrice Vaticana, Vatican City 2005.

———, *Man and Woman He Created Them: A Theology of the Body*, trans. Michael Waldstein, Daughters of St. Paul, Boston 2006.

JOHN XXIII, Encyclical *Mater et Magistra*, 15 May, 1961: in *AAS* 53 (1961): 234–345.

PAUL VI, *Address to Gynaecologists and Obstetricians*, 29 October 1966: *AAS* 58 (1966): 1116–1170.

———, Encyclical *Humanae Vitae*, 25 July 1968: *AAS* 60 (1968): 481–503.

PIUS XI, Encyclical *Casti Connubii*, 31 December 1930: *AAS* 22 (1930): 539–592.

PIUS XII, *Address to the Fourth International Convention of Catholic Doctors*, 29 September 1949: *AAS* 41 (1949): 557–561.

———, *Allocution to Italian Catholic Union of Obstetricians*, 29 October 1951: *AAS* 43 (1951): 835–854.

———, *Allocution to the First Symposium on Genetic Medicine*, 7 September 1953: *AAS* 45 (1953): 596–607.

———, *Address to the Second World on Fertility and Sterility*, 19 May 1956: *AAS* 48 (1953): 467–474.

———, "*Christian Norms of Morality*," 29 September 1949, in The Human Body: Papal Teachings, Monks of Solesmes, (ed.), St. Paul Editions, Daughters of St. Paul, Boston (1960): 117–119.

PONTIFICAL ACADEMY FOR LIFE, *Identity and Statue of Human Embryo: Proceedings of the Third Assembly of the Pontifical Academy for Life*, Juan De Dios Vial Correa and Elio, Sgreccia (eds.), Vatican City, 14–16 February 1997.

———, *The Dignity of Human Procreation and Reproductive Technologies: Anthropological and Ethical Aspects*, Juan De Dios Vial Correa and Elio, Sgreccia (eds.), Liberia Editrice Vaticana, Vatican City 2005.

———, "Communiqué of the Pontifical Academy for Life," in Juan De Dios Vial Correa and Elio, Sgreccia (eds.), *The Dignity of Human Procreation and Reproductive Technologies: Anthropological and Ethical Aspects*, Liberia Editrice Vaticana, Vatican City 2005.

———, *The Human Embryo Before Implantation: Scientific and Bioethical Considerations: Proceedings of the Twelfth Assembly of the Pontifical Academy for Life*, Elio Sgreccia and Jean Laffite (eds.), Vatican City, 27 February 1 March 2006.

SECOND VATICAN COUNCIL: Pastoral Constitution *Gaudium et Spes*, 7 December 1965: in *AAS* 58 (1966): 1025–1115.

Primary Sources

Works on the Simple Case

CAHILL, Lisa Sowle, "The Vatican Document on Bioethics: Two Responses," in *America* 156, 12 (1988): 246–247.

———, "Catholic Sexual Ethics and the Dignity of the Person: A Double Message," in *Theological Studies* 50 (1989): 120–150.

CARLSON, John W., "Interventions upon Gametes in Assisting the Conjugal Act toward Fertilization," in *Philosophy and Medicine* 53 (1989): 107–124.

———, "*Donum Vitae* on Homologous Interventions: Is IVF-ET a Less Acceptable Gift than 'GIFT?'," in *Journal of Medical Philosophy* 14, 5 (1989): 523–540.

COVI, Ettore, "L'istruzione '*Donum vitae*,' e la condanna della FIVET omologa simple case," in *Laurentianum* 28, 1 (1987): 328–356.

DOERFLER, John, *Donum Vitae Twenty Years After: The Debate whether It Is Intrinsically Evil to Generate Human Life by Means other than the Marital Act*, Dissertation, Pontificia Universitas Lateranensis, Pontificium Institutum Joannes Paulus II, Studiorum Matrimonii et Familiae, Rome 2010.

KACZNSKI, Edward, Rispetto per la vita nascente e dignità della procreazione, in *Angelicum, Teologia* 64 (1987): 583–591.

KEENAN, James F., "Moral Horizons in Health Care: Reproductive Technologies and Catholic Identity," in *Philosophy and Medicine* 53 (1989): 53–71.

MAY, William E., "The Simple Case of In Vitro Fertilization and Embryo Transfer," in *Linacre Quarterly* 55, 1 (1988): 29–43.

———, "Catholic Teaching on In Vitro Fertilization," in Donald G. McCarthy (ed.), *Reproductive Technologies, Marriage and the Church*, The Pope John XXIII Medical-Moral Research Center, Braintree, MA (1988): 107–121.

———, "*Donum Vitae*: Catholic Teaching Concerning Homologous In Vitro Fertilization," in *Philosophy and Medicine* 53 (1989): 73–92.

———, *Catholic Bioethics and the Gift of Human Life*, 2nd edition, Our Sunday Visitor, Indiana (2008): 80–90.

MCCORMICK, Richard A., "Document is Unpersuasive," in *Health Progress* 68 (1987): 53–55.

———, "The Vatican Document on Bioethics: Two Responses," in *America* 156, 12 (1987): 247–248.

———, "Therapy or Tampering: The Ethics of Reproductive Technology and the Development of Doctrines," in *The Critical Calling: Reflections on Moral Dilemmas Since Vatican II*, Georgetown University Press, Washington D.C. (1989): 329–352.

PORTER, Jean, "Human Need and Natural Law," in *Philosophy and Medicine* 53 (1989): 93–106.

TAUER, Carol A., "*Donum Vitae*: Dissenting Opinions on the 'Simple Case' of In Vitro Fertilization" in *Philosophy and Medicine* 53 (1989): 125–146.

TONTI-FILIPPINI, Nicholas, "IVF: The Role of the Technician," in Charles Connolly (ed.), *New Life: Catholic Teaching on Technology and Fertilization, with Commentaries*, Four Courts Press, Dublin (1987): 71–74.

Publications on *Donum Vitae*

AMERICAN FERTILITY SOCIETY, ETHICS COMMITTEE (1986–87), "Ethical Considerations of the New Reproductive Technologies, in the Light of Instruction on Respect for Human Life in Its Origin and on the Dignity of Procreation, Issued by the Congregation for the Doctrine of the Faith," in *Fertility and Sterility* 49, 2 (1988): 1–7.

ASCI, Donald P., *The Conjugal Act as a Personal Act: A Study of the Catholic Concept of the Conjugal Act in the Light of Christian Anthropology*, Ignatius Press, San Francisco (2002): 154–163.

BARBÀRA, Emmanuel, *Donum Vitae: Continuity and Development in Church Teaching*, Pontificia Universitas Lateranensis, Academica Alfonsiana, Rome (1994).

BAUZON, Stéphane, "Catholic Reflections for an Updated *Donum Vitae* Instruction: A New Catholic Challenge in a Post-Christian Europe," in *Christian Bioethics* 14, 1 (2008): 42–57.

BERNARDIN, Joseph, "Dignity of Procreation: Science and the Creation of Life," *Origins* 17, 2 (1988): 21–26.

———, "nuevo documento vaticano sobre bioetica," in *Studium* 49 (2009): 3–40.

BERQUIST, Richard, "The Dignity of Human Life and Procreation," in *Crisis* 5, 5 (1987): 24–28.

BIRNBACKER, Dieter, "Gefährdet die Moderne Reproduktionsmedizin die Menschliche Würde?" in *Information Philosophie* (1989): 5–15.

BOYLE, Joseph. "An Introduction to the Vatican Instruction on Reproductive Technologies," in *Linacre Quarterly* 55, 1 (1988): 20–8.

———, (ed.), *Creative Love: The Ethics of Human Reproduction*, Christendom Press, Front Royal, VA (1989).

BRIANCESCO, Eduardo, "Una lectura teológica de la instrucción romana '*donum vitae*,'" in *Teologia* 25 (1988): 71–91.

BYK, Christian, "*Donum Vitae*: Civil Law and Moral Values," in *The Journal of Medicine and Philosophy* 14, 5 (1989): 561–73.

CAHILL, Lisa Sowle, "Moral Traditions, Ethical Language, and Reproductive Technologies," in *Journal of Medicine and philosophy* 14, 5 (1989): 497–522.

———, "What is the Nature of the Unity of Sex, Love and Procreation? A Response to Elio Sgreccia," in Edmund D. Pellegrino, John Collins Harvey and John P. Langan (eds.), *Gift of Life: Catholic Scholars Respond to the Vatican Instruction*, Georgetown University Press, Washington D.C. (1990): 137–148.

CHAPELLE, Albert, Pour lire '*Donum vitae*,'" in *Nouvelle Revue Théologique* 109, 4 (1987): 481–508.

COLLINS, Harvey J., "Diagnosing the Vatican 'Instruction,'" in *Commonweal* 114, 8 (1987): 239.

———, "Speculations Regarding the History of *Donum Vitae*," in *The Journal of Medicine and Philosophy* 14, 5 (1989): 481–491.

COLLITON, William F. Jr., "In Vitro Fertilization and the Wisdom of the Catholic Church," in *Linacre Quarterly* 74 (2007): 10–29.

CONNOLLY, Charles (ed.), *New Life: Church Teaching on Technology and Fertilization*, Four Courts Press, Dublin (1987).

COX, Kathryn Lilla, "Toward a Theology of Infertility and the Role of *Donum Vitae*," in *Horizons* 40, 1 (2013): 28–52.

DALY, Thomas V., *Life and Sex are Good: An Introductory Comment on Donum Vitae*, Ares, Milano (1988).

DANIEL, William, "Towards a Theology of Procreation: An Examination of the Vatican Instruction *Donum Vitae*," in *Pacifica* 3 (1990): 61–86.

DELADURANTAYE, Paul F., "From *Humanae Vitae* to *Donum Vitae*: Symmetry and Consistency in Catholic Biomedical Teaching," in *The Linacre Quarterly* 66, 1 (1999): 7–20.

DE LA NOI, Pedro, "Análisis filosófico de la instrucción sobre el respeto de la vida nasciente y la dignidad de la procreación," in *Teologia y Vida* 21, 1 (1988): 25–38.

DOERFLER, John, "In Vitro Fertilization and the Person," in *Ethics and Medics* 25, 5 (2000): 3–4.

DUCHARME, Howard M., "The Vatican's Dilemma: On the Morality of IVF and the Incarnation," in *Bioethics* 5, 1 (1991): 57–66.

FLEMMING, John L., "A critical Evaluation of the Vatican Instruction on Respect for Human Life," in *Linacre Quarterly* 55, 1 (1988): 13–19.

GAFO, Javier, "Reproduccion humana asistida," in Marciano Vidal (ed.), *conceptos fundamentales de ética teológica,* Editorial Trotta, S.A, Madrid (1992): 493–515.

GIUNCHEDI, Francesco, "Considerazioni sul documento '*Donum vitae*,'" in *Rassegna di Teologia* 28, 3 (1987): 217–229.

GORDON, Gregory W., *Donum Vitae As Donum Nuptiale: The "Instruction on Respect for Human Life in Its Origin and the Dignity of Procreation" in the Immediate Preparation for the Celebration of the Sacrament of Matrimony*, Washington, D.C. (1991).

HABER, Richard, *An Ethical Analysis of Donum Vitae in the Light of Its Commentaries*, Université de Montréal, Montréal (1994).

HARVEY, John Collins, "A Doctor Reflects upon *Donum Vitae*," in *Catholic Medical Quarterly* 39 (1988): 25–32.

———, "Speculations Regarding the History of *Donum Vitae*," in *The Journal of Medicine and Philosophy* 14, 5 (1989): 481–91.

HENNING, Alyssa; RAUCHER, Michal and ZOLOTH, Laurie, "A Jewish Response to the Vatican?" in *The American Journal of Bioethics* 9, 11 (2009): 37–39.

HILPERT, Konrad, "Nach dem Erscheinen der Instruktion *Dignitas Personae*: Zehn Merkmale einer Künftigen Moralverkündigung im Geist der Ermutigung und des Vertrauens," in *Stimmen der Zeit* 227 (2009): 321–335.

HUNT, George W., "New Vatican Instruction on Human Life and Procreation," in *America* 156, 12 (1987): 245.

JOHNSTONE, Brian V., "The Instruction *Donum Vitae* and Its Reception," in *Studia Moralia* 26 (1988): 209–229.

KIELY, Bartholomew, "L'istruzione *'Donum Vitae'*: una reflessione introduttiva," in *La Civilta Catholica* 138, 2 (1987): 11, 22.

———, "Contraception, In Vitro Fertilization and the Principle of Inseparability," in *Humanae Vitae: 20 anni dopo: atti del congresso internazionale di teologia morale* (Roma 9–12 novembre 1988), Edizioni Ares, Milano (1989): 329–336.

KLODKOWSKA, Danuta, *Le document romain "Donum vitae" (1987) sur les nouvelles technologies de procréation*, Université de Montréal, Montréal 1997.

KREIML, Josef, "Humanität im Widerstreit mit der Technik? Die Aussagen der Instruktion *Donum Vitae* zur frage der In-vitro-Befruchtung," in *Forum Kath. Theol.* 6 (1990): 103–116.

LACADENA, Juan-Ramón, "Instrucción *Dignitas Personae* sobre algunas cuestiones de bioética: una puesta al día de la *Donum Vitae*," in *Moralia* 32 (2009): 41–68.

LARIVIERE, Robert Dean, *A Critique of the Instruction on Respect for Human Life in Its Origin and on the Dignity of Procreation, in Relation to Catholic Revisionist Moral Theology*, Catholic University of America, Washington, D.C. (1989).

LEGA, Carlo, "Reflessi giuridici e deontologici nella istruzione sui l rispetto della vita umana nascente e la dignita della procreazione'" in *Medicine e Morale* 37, 5 (1987): 799–816.

LEHMANN, Karl, "Observations sur l'interpretation de l'instruction *Donum Vitae*," in *La Documentation Catholique* 84, 1938 (1987): 431.

LEONE, Salvino, La FIVET omologa nell'istruzione' su questioni bioetiche," in *Rivista di Teologia Morale* 19, 75 (1987): 315–324.

LIPTAK, David Q. and DUFFY, Leo T., *The Gift of Life: A Theological Commentary on the "Instruction on respect for Human life in Its Origin and on the Dignity of Human Procreation: Replies to Certain Questions of the Day,"* Liturgical Publications, Lake Worth (1988).

LÓPEZ, Eduardo A., "El respeto a la vida humana y la dignidad de la procreación," in *Sal Terrae* 75, 4 (1987): 47–59.

LORENZETTI, Luigi, "Etica e techniche bio-mediche: criteri di lettura del documento Ratzinger," in *Rivista di Teologia Morale* 19, 74 (1987): 83–88.

MAGUIRE, Marjorie R., "The Vatican Has Gone Too Far," in *Conscience* 8, 3 (1987): 14–15.

MCCORMICK, Richard A., "The Vatican Document on Bioethics: Some Unsolicited Suggestions," in *America* 156 (1987): 24–28.

MICHALK, Maria, *10 Jahre Donum Vitae Sachsen: ein Resümee*, Weimer, Bertuch, Frankfurt (2010).

MIGLIETTA, Guido M., *Respect for Human Life in Its Origin and the Dignity of Procreation: The Congregation for the Doctrine of the Faith's Instruction "Donum Vitae,"*: An Appraisal, Asti: TSG S.R.L Arti Graphiche (1998).

MOONEN, C.H., "Zu den Assagen der Instruktion vom 22. Februar 1987 über die Künstliche Befruchtung," *ZKT, Teologia* 111 (1989): 197–203.

MORINIERE, Jean and MORINIERE, Jacqueline, "La FIVETE homologue: procréation limitée, procréation assistée dan un couple: le point de vue d'un couple de médicins catholiques," in *Le Supplément* 177 (1991): 67–75.

OVERDUIN, Daniel C., "A Response to the Vatican Document on IVF and Related Issues," in *Lutheran Theological Journal* 21, 2 (1987): 82–89.

PAOLINELLI, Marco, "Natura umana e persona umana: la dignità della procreazione: Il fascino della tecnica e la domanda umana," in *Medicina e Morale* 37, 3 (1987): 5–12.

PELLEGRINO, Edmund, D. and HARVEY, John C. and LANGAN, John P. (eds.), *Gift of Life: Catholic Scholars Respond to the Vatican Instruction*, Georgetown University Press, Washington, D.C. (1990).

PERICO, Giacomo, "L'istruzione vaticana *Donum vitae*: lettura e annotazioni," in *Aggiornamenti Sociali* 38, 6 (1987): 977–985.

PÉREZ SÁNCHEZ, Alfredo, "Instrucción sobre el respeto de la vida humana nasciente y la dignidad de la procreación, respuesta a algunas cuestiones de actualidad," in *Teologia y Vida* 29, 1 (1987): 5–12.

RHONHEIMER, Martin, *Ethics of Procreation and the Defense of Human Life: Contraception, Artificial Fertilization and Abortion*, edited by William F. Murphy Jr., The Catholic University of America Press, Washington, D.C. (2010): 153–227.

RIGA, Peter J., "The Vatican's Instruction on Human Life," in *Linacre Quarterly* 54, 3 (1987): 16–21.

RUINI, Camillo, "L'immagine della famiglia nel documento 'il dono della vita,'" in *Medicina e Morale* 37, 6 (1987): 977–985.

SEIFERT, Josef, "Substituting or Replacing the Conjugal Act or Assistance to It? IVF, GIFT and Some Other Medical Interventions, Philosophical Reflections on the Vatican Declaration *Donum Vitae*," in *Anthropotes* 4 (1988): 273–286.

SELLING, Joseph A., "The Instruction on Respect for Life: II. Dealing with the Issues," in *Louvain Studies* 12 (1987): 323–361.

SGRECCIA, Elio, "Moral Theology and Artificial Procreation in Light of *Donum Vitae*," in Edmund D. Pellegrino, John Collins Harvey and John P. Langan (eds.), *Gift of Life: Catholic Scholars Respond to the Vatican Instruction*, Georgetown University Press, Washington D.C. (1990): 115–135.

———, (ed.), *Il dono della vita: istruzione della congregazione per la dottrina della fede su il respetto della vita umana nascente e la dignitá della procreazione umana*, Edizione Vita e Pensiero, Milano (1987).

SHANNON, Thomas A. and CAHILL, Lisa S. (eds.), *Religion and Artificial Reproduction: An Inquiry into the Vatican Instruction on Respect for Human Life*, Crossroad, New York (1988).

SHEETS, John, "Christian Anthropology as It Applies to Reproductive and Sexual Morality," in Marilyn Wallace and Thomas Hilgers (eds.), *The Gift of Life: Proceedings of a National Conference on the Vatican Instruction on Reproductive Ethics and Technology*, Pope Paul VI Institute Press, Omaha, NE (1990): 177–191.

SHÜLLER, Bruno, "Paraenesis and Moral Argument in *Donum Vitae*," in Edmund Pellegrino and Collins Harvey (eds.), *Gift of Life: Catholic Scholars Respond to the Vatican Instruction*, Georgetown University Press, Washington, D.C. (1990): 82–98.

SMITH, Janet E., "The Introduction to the Vatican Instruction," in Donald McCarthy (ed.), *Reproductive Technologies, Marriage and the Church*, Pope John XIII Medical-Moral Research and Education Center, Braintree, MA (1988): 13–28.

SPAEMANN, Robert, "Kommentar zur Instruktion *Donum Vitae*," in Die Unantastbarkeit des menschlichen Lebens, Zu ethischen Fragen der

Biomedizin, Instruktion der Kongregation für die Glaubenslehre. Mit einem Kommentar von R. Spaemann. Herder Verlag, Freiburg (1987).

TESTART, Jacques, "Procréations medicalment assistées: l'ethique et la loi," in *Études* 381 (1994): 399–610.

TONTI-FILIPPINI, Nicholas, "'*Donum Vitae*' and Gamete Intra-Fallopian Tube Transfer," in *Linacre Quarterly* 57, 2 (1989): 68–79.

UNITED STATES CONFERENCE OF BISHOPS, *Ethical and Religious Directives for Catholic Health Care Services*, 5th edition, USCCB, Washington, D.C. (2009).

—— (ed.), *Instruction Donum Vitae: Commentaries and Studies Series*, Libreria Editrice Vaticana, Washington, D.C. (2013).

VACEK, Edward V., "Vatican Instruction on Reproductive Technology," in *Theological Studies* 49 (1988): 110–131.

VESPIEREN, Patrick, "Les fécondations artificielles: a propos de l'instruction romaine sur 'le don de la vie,'" in *Études* 366, 5 (1987): 607–619.

VIDAL, Marciano, ELIZARI, Javier and RUBIO, Miguel, *El don de la vida: etica de la procreacíon humana*, Editorial Covarrubias, Grafinat, S.A., Madrid (1987).

——, "'El don de la vida': comentarios teológico-morales a la instrucción de la santa sede," in *Moralia* 9, 3–4 (1987).

WALLACE, Marilyn and HILGERS, Thomas (eds.), *The Gift of Life: The Proceedings of a National Conference on the Vatican Instruction on Reproductive Ethics and Technology*, Pope Paul VI Institute Press, Omaha, NE (1990).

WEHOWSKY, Stephan (ed.), *Lebensbeginn und Menschlich Würde: Stellungnahmen zur Instrucktion der Kongregation für die Glaubenslehre vom 22.2.1987*, (Gentechnologie: Chancen und Risiken, 14) Frankfurt am Main, München (1987): x-166.

Secondary Sources

Theological Works on In Vitro Fertilization

Aa. Vv., "Journal of In Vitro Fertilization and Embryo Transfer: IVF," in *Journal of In Vitro Fertilization and Embryo Transfer: IVF*, New York (1984).

ANSALDI, Jean, "Ethical Considerations of the New Reproductive Technologies." in *Fertility and Sterility* 46, 3 (1986): 1S–94S.

———, "Anthropologie et fécundation in vitro: une éthique sous la croix," in *ÈTR* 64, 5 (1989): 45–57.

AUGENSTEIN, Leroy, *Come Let Us Play God*, Harper and Row Publishers, New York (1969).

BARRAGAN, Lozano J., "Some Biblical Signs on Human Procreation" in Juan De Dios Vial C. and Elio Sgreccia (eds.), *The dignity of Human Procreation and Reproductive Technologies: Anthropological and Ethical Aspects*, Liberia Vaticana, Vatican City (2005): 21–32.

BARTELS, Dianne M. (ed. et al.), *Beyond Baby Making: Ethical Issues in New Reproductive Technologies*, Humana Press, New Jersey (1990).

BELLIOTTI, Raymond A., "Morality And In Vitro Fertilization," in *Bioethics Quarterly* 2 (1980): 6–19.

BERNADIN, Joseph, "Science and the Creation of Human Life: Responses to the Vatican Document of Reproductive Technologies," in *Catholic Health Association, St. Louis*, Washington, D.C. (1987): 3–6.

BIRNBACHER, Dieter, Gefährdet die Moderne Reproduktionsmedizin die Menschlich Würde? In Volkmar Braun (Ed. et al.), *Ethische und Rechtliche Fragen de Gentechnologie und der Reproduktionsmedizin* (1987): 77–88.

BLANK, Robert H., "Making Babies: The State of the Art," in *Futurist* 19 (1985): 11–7.

BLÁZQUEZ, Niceto, "Bioetica y dignidad de la procreacion humana," in *Studium* 28, 1 (1988): 35–65.

BOMPIANI, Andriano, "Gli aspetti tecnici della fecondation in vitro e dell'embryo transfer umano," in *Federation Medica* 37, 1 (1984): 5–13.

BRUGGER, Christian E., "In Defense of the Morality of Transferring Heterologous Embryos," in *National Catholic Bioethics Quarterly* 5,1 (2005): 95–112.

BRUGUÈS, Jean-Louis, "La F.I.V.E.T.E. au risque de l'ethique chrétienne," in *Revue Thomiste* 87 (1987): 45–83.

———, *La fécondation artificielle: au crible de l'éthique chrétienne*, Fayard, Paris (1989).

———, *Fecondatione artificiale: una scelta etica?* Trans. Maura Vecchietti, Socità Editrice Internationale, Torino (1991).

BYK, Christian (ed.), *Procreation artificielle ou en sont l'ethique et le droite? une contribution uultidisciplinaire et internationale*, Editions Alesandre Lacassagne, Lyon (1989).

CAFFARRA, Carlo, "The Moral Problem of Artificial Insemination," in *Linacre Quarterly* 55 (1988): 37–43.

CAHILL, Lisa Sowle, "In Vitro Fertilization: Ethical Issues in Judaeo-Christian Perspective," in *Loyola Law Review* 32 (1986): 337.

———, "Women, Marriage, Parenthood: What Are Their 'Natures'?" in *Logos* 9, 1 (1988): 11–35.

CALLAHAN, Sidney, "The Ethical Challenge of the New Reproductive Technology," in M. Therese Lysaught and Joseph J. Kotva Jr. (ed. et al.) *On Moral Medicine: Theological Perspectives in Medical Ethics*, 3rd edition, Grand Rapids, Cambridge (2012): 858–864.

CATALDO, Peter, "The Newest Reproductive Technologies: Applying Catholic Teaching," in Russell Smith (ed.) *The Gospel of Life and the Vision of Health Care*, The Pope John XXIII Medical Centre, Braintree, MA (1996): 61–94.

———, "Reproductive Technologies," in *Ethics and Medics* 21 (1996): 1–3.

CHERVENAK, Frank A., MCCULLOUGH, Laurence B. and ROSENWAKS, Zev, "Ethical Dimensions of the Number of Embryos to Be Transferred in In Vitro Fertilization," in *Journal of Assisted Reproduction and Genetics* 18, 11 (2001): 583–587.

COHEN, Cynthia B., "Give Me Children or I Shall Die!: New Reproductive Technologies and Harm to Children," in *The Hastings Center Report* 26, 2 (1996): 19–27.

COHEN, Mark E., "The 'Brave New Baby' and the Law: Fashioning Remedies for the Victims of in Vitro Fertilization," in *American Journal of Law and Medicine* 4 (1978): 319.

COLEMAN, Stephen, *The Ethics of Artificial Uteruses: Implications for Reproduction and Abortion*, Ashgate Publishing Company, Burlington (2004).

COLLIN, Russel, *Human Embryos: Debate on Assisted Reproduction*, Oxford University Press, New York (1989).

CONOLLY, Charles (ed.). *New Life: Church Teaching on Technology and Fertilization, With Commentaries*, Four Courts Press, Dublin (1987).

CURRAN, Charles, *Issues in Sexual and medical Ethics*, University of Notre Dame Press, Indiana (1978).

———, *Change in Official Catholic Moral Teachings*, Paulist Press, New York (2003).

CURRAN, Charles and MCCORMICK, Richard A. (eds.), *Readings in Moral Theology: Moral Norms and the Catholic Tradition*, Paulist Press, New York (1979).

DEMARCO, Donald T., *Infertility and In Vitro Fertilization: Its Meaning and Morality*, Life Ethics Centre, St. Joseph's University College, Edmonton, Alta (1985).

DE ROSA, Francis M., "In Vitro Fertilization and the Person," in *Ethics and Medics* 25, 5 (2000): 3–4.

DOERFLER, John, *Assisting or Replacing the Conjugal Act: Criteria for a Moral Evaluation of Reproductive Techniques*, Unpublished S.T.L Dissertation on file at the John Paul II *Institute for Studies on Marriage and Family*, Washington, D.C. (1999).

DUNSTAN, Gerbert R., "The Ethical, Scientific and Medical Implications of Human Conception In Vitro," in *Modern Biological Experimentation*, Città del Vaticano (1984): 193–249.

———, "In-vitro Fertilization: The Ethics," in *Human Reproduction* (1986): 41–44.

———, "The Bumpy Road to Human In Vitro Fertilization," in *Nature Medicine* 7, 10 (2001): 1091–1094.

DYSON, Anthony, *The Ethics of IVF*, Mowbray, New York (1995).

EDWARDS, Robert G., "Fertilization of Human Eggs In Vitro: Morals, Ethics and the Law," in *Quarterly Review Bioethics* 49 (1974): 3–26.

EDWARDS, Richard G. and STEPTOE, Patrick, *A Matter of Life*, William Morrow and Co., New York (1980).

EVANS, Debra, *Without Moral Limits: Women, Reproduction, and Medical Technology*, Crossway, Wheaton (2000).

FEINBERG, John S. and Feinberg, Paul D., *Ethics for a Brave New World*, Crossway, Wheaton, Illinois (2010).

FERRE, Jorge J. and DE ARTOLA, Martínez V., "Fecundación artificial: aspetos mèdicos y cuestiones," in *Revista de Medicina de la Universidad de Navarra*, 29, 3 (1995): 201–206.

FLEMING, John I., *Dignitas Personae Explained: A Catholic Church's Teaching on Reproductive and Related Technologies*, Connor Court Publishing, Herefordshire (2010).

FRALING, Bernhard, "Ethisch-theologische Bewertung der Extrakorporalen Befruchtung," *Theol. Und Glaube*, t. 75 (1985): 269–285.

FRAME, Tom R., *Alternative Parenthood: The Ethics of Defying Nature*, University of New South Wales Press, Sydney (2008).

FRANCOUER, Robert, *Adam's Rib*, New York Hardcourt Brace, New York (1972).

———, *Utopian Motherhood, New Trends in Human Reproduction*, A. S. Barnes and Co., New York (1973).

FREDERICKS, Christopher M., PAULSON, John D. and DECHERNEY, Alan H., *Foundations of In Vitro Fertilization*, Hemisphere Publication, Washington (1987).

FULLICK, Ann, *In Vitro Fertilization*, Heinemann Library, Oxford (2002).

FUNGHI, Patrizia, *Bioetica e cattolicesimo: quale e la liceità dell'intervento scientifico sulla vita umana?*, *Atheneum*, Firenze (1993).

GARCÍA DE HARO, R., "La fecondazione artificiale," in *Studi Cattolici* 278, 279 (1984): 269–274.

GELFAND, Scot and SHOOK, John R. (eds.), *Ectogenesis: Artificial Womb Technology and the Future of Human Reproduction*, Editions Rodopi B.V, New York (2006).

GEMELLI, A., *La fecondazione artificiale*, Vita and Pensiero, Milano (1949).

GERBER, Rona, "In Vitro Fertilization, AID and Embryo-experimentation: Some Moral Considerations," in *Journal of Applied Philosophy* 3, 1 (1986): 103–109.

GIUNCHEDI, Filippo, "La FIVET: opinioni teologico-morali," in *Rivista Teologia Morale*, t. 19, 73 (1987): 57–65.

HAAS, John M., "The Inseparability of the Two Meanings of the Marriage Act," in Donald McCarthy (ed.), *Reproductive Technologies, Marriage, and the Church*, Pope John XIII Medical- Moral Research and Education Center, Braintree, MA (1988), 89–106.

HALL, Theodore, "Test Tube Babies and Beyond: Moral Considerations," in *Homiletical Pastoral Review* 79, 5 (1979): 25–32.

HANDWERKER, Lisa, "Social and Ethical Implications of in Vitro Fertilization in Contemporary China," in *Cambridge Quarterly of Healthcare Ethics* 4, 3 (1995): 355–363.

HARRIS, John, "In Vitro Fertilization: The Ethical Issues (I)," in *The Philosophical Quarterly* 33, 132 (1983): 217–237.

HEITMAN, Elizabeth, "Social and Ethical Aspects of In Vitro Fertilization," in *International Journal of Technology Assessment in Health Care*, 15, 1 (1999): 22–35.

HELLEGERS, André E. and MCCORMICK, Richard A., "Unanswered Questions on Test Tube Life," in *America* 139, 4 (1978): 12–19.

HUXLEY, Aldous, *Brave New World*, Harper Torch, New York (1960).

JAMES, David N., "Artificial Insemination: A Reexamination," in *Philosophy and Theology* 2, 4 (1988): 305–26.

JONES, Howard W., "The Ethics of In Vitro Fertilization," in *Fertility and Sterility* 37, 1 (1982): 146–149.

KAEBNICK, Gregory E. and Murray, Thomas H. (eds.), *Synthetic Biology and Morality: Artificial Life and the Bounds of Nature*, MIT Press, Massachusetts (2013).

KASS, Leon R., "Babies by Means of In Vitro Fertilization: Unethical Experiments on the Unborn?" in *The New England Journal of Medicine* 285, 21 (1971): 1174.

———, "'Making Babies' Revisited," in *Public Interest* 54 (1979): 32–60.

KRAUTHERMMER, Charles, "The Ethics of Human Manufacture," in *New Republic* 196, 18 (1987): 17–21.

LAURITZEN, Paul, "Whose Bodies? Which Selves? Appeals to Embodiment in Assessments of Reproductive Technology," in Lysaught, M. Therese and Kotva Joseph J. Jr. (eds. et al.) *On Moral Medicine: Theological Perspectives in Medical Ethics*, 3rd edition, Grand Rapids, Cambridge (2012): 846–857.

MACHEREL, Jeanne and Oliver, "Stérilité pour le vie: confrontes à des traitment astreignants," in *Études* 366, 5 (1987): 62–625.

MACKLIN, Ruth, "Ethical Issues in the New Reproductive Technology," in *Journal of Reproductive Health, Rights and Ethics* 3 (1997): 69–85.

MCCARTAN, Karen M., "A Survey of the Legal, Ethical, and Public Policy Considerations of In Vitro Fertilization," in *Notre Dame JL Ethics & Public Policy* 2 (1985): 695.

MCCARTHY, Joseph J., "In Vitro Technology: A Threat to the Covenant," in *Health Program* 68, 2 (1987): 44–8.

MCCORMICK, Richard A., The Ethical and Religious Challenges of Reproductive Technology, in *Cambridge Quarterly of Healthcare Ethics* 8, 4 (1999): 547–556.

MELINA, Livio, *Corso di bioetica: Il vangelo della vita*, Edizione Piemme, Milano (1996).

———, "The Intrinsic Logic of Interventions in the Field of Human Artificial Procreation: Ethical Aspects," in Juan De Dios Vial Correa and Elio Sgreccia (eds.), *The Dignity of Human Procreation and Reproductive Technologies: Anthropological and Ethical Aspects*, Liberia Vaticana, Vatican City (2005): 114–126.

MELO-MARTIN, De Immaculata, *Making Babies: Biomedical Technologies, Reproductive Ethics, and Public Policy*, Kluwer Academic, Dordrecht; Boston (1998).

O'ROURKE, Kevin D., "Catholic Principles and In Vitro Fertilization," in *National Catholic Bioethics Quarterly* 10, 4 (Winter 2010): 709–722.

PADILLA, Montecillo F., *The Morality of Human In Vitro Fertilization: Its Impact on Marriage, Family and Society Based on the Teaching of Pius XII and Paul VI*, Dissertation, Pontificia Studiorum Universitas a S. Thoma Aq. in Urbe, Rome (1983).

PARKER, Steve, *In Vitro Fertilization*, World Almanac Library, Milwaukee, WI (2007).

PEREGO, Angelo, *La fecondazione umana in vitro e la sua problematica morale e teologica*, Paedeia, Brescia (1964).

PRIVITERA, Salvatore, "In Vitro Befruchtung: die Argumentation der Moral Theologie," in *Theol. Und Glaube, Teologia* 77 (1987): 291–300.

RAMSEY, Paul, *The Fabricated Man*, Yale University Press, London (1970).

———, "Shall We 'Reproduce'?" in *The Journal of the American Medical Association* 220, 10 (1972): 1346–1350.

———, "Shall We 'Reproduce'? II. Rejoinders and Future Forecast," in *Journal of the American Medical Association* 220, 11 (1972): 1480–1485.

REIBER, David T., "The Morality of Artificial Womb Technology," in *The Catholic Bioethics Quarterly* 10, 3 (2010): 515–527.

REICH, Warren T., "Ethical Issues in In Vitro Fertilization and Fetal Experimentation," *Videotape*, Rochester: Nazareth College of Rochester, April 4–6, 1979.

RHOLEDER, Hermann, *Test-Tube Babies*, Panurge Press, New York (1974).

RICHIE, Cristina, "Applying Catholic Responsibility to In Vitro Fertilization: Obligations to the Spouse, the Body, and the Common Good," in *Christian Bioethics* 18, 3 (2012): 271–286.

ROBERTS, Elizabeth F. S., "God's Laboratory: Religious Rationalities and Modernity in Ecuadorian In Vitro Fertilization," in *Culture, Medicine and Psychiatry* 30, 4 (2006): 507–536.

RODRÍGUEZ-LUÑO, Ángel, and LÓPEZ Mondéjar R., *La fecondazione in vitro: aspetti medici e morali*, Città Nuova, Roma (1986).

RÖMELT, Josef, "Theologische Ethik und In-Vitro-Fertilisation," in *Studia Moralia* 37 (1999): 357–370.

RORVICK, David, *Brave New Baby*, Doubleday and Co., New York (1969).

SCHLAG, Martin, "In-Vitro Fertilisation und Lebensrecht," in *IMABE-Institut/Schweizerische Gesellschaft für Bioethik (Hg), Der Status des Embryos*, Wien (1989): 117ff.

———, *Verfassungsrechtliche Aspekte der Künstlichen Fortpflanzung. Insbesondere das Lebensrecht des in vitro gezeugten Embryos*, Braumüller-Verlag, Wien (1991).

SCHOCKENHOFF, Eberhard, *Ethik Des Lebens: Grundlagen und Neue Herausforderungen*, Herder, Freiburg (2009).

SHANNON, Thomas A., "In Vitro Fertilization: Ethical Issues," in *Women and Health* 13, 1–2 (1988): 155–165.

———, *The Nature and Dignity of the Human Person as the Foundation of the Right to Life: The Challenges of the Contemporary Cultural Context*, Libreria Editrice Vaticana, Vatican City (2002).

SHER, Geoffrey, DAVIS, Virginia Marriage and STOESS, Jean, "Ethical Issues Involved with in Vitro Fertilization," in *AORN Journal* 52, 3 (1990): 627–631.

———, *In Vitro Fertilization: The A.R.T. of Making Babies*, 3rd edition, Facts on File, Inc., New York (1995).

SPRINGER, Robert H., "Notes on Moral Theology: Sterilization and Artificial Insemination," in *Theological Studies* 31, 3 (1970): 507–509 (476–5211).

STUDDARD, Albert, "The Morality of in Vitro Fertilization," in *Human Life Review* 5, 4 (1979): 41–55.

SUAREZ, Antoine, "Darf man dem Embryo den verfassundgrechtlichen Schutz der Menscenwürde absprechen?, in *Schweizerische Juristenzeitung* 86 (1990): 205–2011.

———, "Gedanken über die Individualität des Menschlichen Frühembyos, Schweizerischen Gesellschaft für Bioethik," in *Lausanne, Sesión del día* 28-19-86.

TAUER, Carol A., "In Vitro fertilization: Are there still Ethical Problems?" in *Journal of the Minnesota Academy of Science* 54, 3 (1989): 3–7.

———, "Essential Ethical Considerations for Public Policy on Assisted Reproduction," in Dianne, M. Bartels (et al.), *Beyond Baby Making*, Humana Press, Clifton, New Jersey (1990): 65–86.

TETTAMANZI, Dionigi, "Louise Brown: la fecundazione artificiale e acune considerazioni morali," in *Anime e Corpi* 15, 78 (1978): 399–418.

———, "Problemi etici sulla fertilizzazione in vitro e sull'embryo transfer," in *Medicina e Morale* 33, 4 (1983): 342–364.

———, "Gli interventi del magistero della chiesa sulla fecondazione in vitro" in *La Scuola Catholica* 113, 1 (1985): 67–113.

———, "Il procreare umano e la fecondazione in vitro, considerationi anthropologiche e etiche," in *Medicina e Morale* 36, 2 (1986): 347–367.

———, "responsabili del dono della vita," in *Anime e Corpi* 26, 146 (1989): 609–244.

VEGA, Gutiérrez A. M., fecundación artificial y ética: cómo formular un judicio ético con validez cientifíca?" in *Moralia, t.* 7 (1985): 16–21.

———, "Ética, legalidad y familia en las técnicas de reproducción humana assisda," in *Ius Canonicum* 35 (1995): 673–728.

WAKEFIELD, John C., *Artful Childmaking: Artificial Insemination in Catholic Teaching*, The Pope John XXIII Medical-Moral Research and Education Center, St. Louis, Missouri (1978).

WALTERS, LeRoy, "Ethics and New Reproductive Technologies: An International Review of Committee Statements," *Hastings Centre Report* 17 (Spec. Supp. June, 1987): 3–9.

WALTERS, William A.W. and SINGER, Peter, *Test-tube Babies: A Guide to Moral Questions, Present Techniques, and Future Possibilities*, Oxford University Press, Oxford (1982).

WOLF, Don P. and QUIGLEY, Martin M., *Human In Vitro Fertilization and Embryo Transfer,* Plenum Press, New York (1984).

YAVARONE, Mark, "In Vitro Fertilization: Truth and Consequences," in *The Linacre Quarterly* 66, 4 (1999): 79–88.

General Theological Works

ALTMAN, Linda J., *Bioethics: Who Lives, Who Dies, and Who Decides?* Enslow Publishers, New Jersey (2006).

ARCHARD, David and BENATAR, David, *Procreation and Parenthood: The Ethics of Bearing Children*, Oxford University Press, New York (2010).

ASCI, Donald P., *The Conjugal Act as a Personal Act: A Study of the Catholic Concept of the Conjugal Act in the Light of Christian Anthropology*, Ignatius Press, San Francisco (2002).

BARUCH, Elaine H. and D'ADAMO, Amadeo Jr. (eds. et al.), *Embryos, Ethics, and Women's Rights: Exploring the New Reproductive Technologies,* Psychology Press, New York (1988).

BEHENKE, John, *Challenging Biomedical Problems: Directions Toward Their Solutions*, Oxford University Press, New York (1972).

BENEDICT, Ashley, O'ROURKE, Kevin D. and DEBLOIS, Jean, *Health Care Ethics*, 5th edition, Georgetown University press, Washington, D.C. (2005).

BENEGIANO, Giuseppe, SABINA, Carrara, and VALENTINA, Filippi, "Robert G Edwards and the Roman Catholic Church," in *Reproductive Biomedicine Online* 22, 7 (2011): 665–672.

BONNICKSEN, Andrea L., *In Vitro Fertilization: Building Policy from Laboratories to Legislatures*, Columbia University Press, New York (1989).

BONNOR, Alfonsus, *Medicine and Man*, Burns and Oates, London (1965).

BOTKIN, Jeffrey R., "Ethical Issues and Practical Problems in Pre-implantation Genetic Diagnosis," in *The Journal of Law, Medicine & Ethics* 26 (1998): 17–28.

BROSENS, Ivo (ed.), *The Challenge of Reproductive Medicine at the Catholic Universities*, Peeters Publishers, Leuven (2006).

BRUNGARDT, Gerard S., "The Face of the Other: Why We Treat the Human Person Differently," in *Journal of Medicine and the Person* 9 (2011): 13–16.

CALLAHAN, Daniel, "Bioethics and Fatherhood," in *Utah Law Review* 3 (1992): 735–746.

CATALDO, Peter, "Reproductive Technologies," in *Ethics and Medics* 2 (1996): 1–3.

CHESHIRE, William P. and JONES, Nancy L., "Can Artificial Techniques Supply Morally Neutral Human Embryos for Research?" in *Ethics and Medicine* 21, 2 (2005): 73–88.

CLARKE, Morgan, "New Kinship, Islam, and the Liberal Tradition: Sexual Morality and New Reproductive Technology in Lebanon," in *Journal of the Royal Anthropological Institute* 14, 1 (2008): 153–169.

COLLIN, Russell Austin, *Human Embryos: The Debate on Assisted Reproduction, Oxford University Press*, Oxford-Tokyo (1989).

CORKERY, Pádraig, *Bioethics and the Catholic Moral Tradition*, Veritas Publications, Dublin (2010).

EBERL, Jason T., "The Beginning of Personhood: A Thomistic Biological Analysis," in *Bioethics* 14, 2 (2000): 134–157.

DOBZHANSKY, Theodosius, *Mankind Evolving*, Bentam Books, Matrix Edition, New York (1970).

DOERFLER, John, "Technology and Human Reproduction," in *Ethics and Medics* 24,8 (1999): 3–4.

EVANS, Donald and PICKERING, Neil, *Creating the Child: The Ethics, Law and Practice of Assisted Reproduction*, Martinus Nijhhoff Publishers, Boston (1996).

FAGOT-LAREGEAULT, Anne, "Reproductive Technology: In France, Debate and Indecision," in *The Hastings Center Report* 17, 3 (1987): 10–12.

FRANCOUER, Robert, *Adam's Rib*, New York Hardcourt Brace, New York (1972).

———, *Utopian Motherhood, New Trends in Human Reproduction*, A. S. Barnes and Co., New York (1973).

GLAZEBROOK, Peter R., Human Beginnings, in *The Cambridge Law Journal* 43, 2 (1984): 209–214.

GRISEZ, Germain, *The Way of the Lord Jesus, Living a Christian Life*, Vol. 2, Franciscan Press, Quincy, IL (1993).

———, *The Way of the Lord Jesus: Difficult Moral Questions*, Vol. 3, Franciscan Press, Quincy, IL (1997).

HANEN, Marsha P. and NIELSEN, Kai, *Science, Morality and Feminist Theory*, University of Calgary Press, Calgary, Alta (1987).

HANMER, Jalna, "Reproduction Trends and the Emergence of Moral Panic," in *Social Science and Medicine* 25, 6 (1987): 697–704.

HESTER, Michael D., "Reproductive Technologies as Instruments of Meaningful Parenting: Ethics in the Age of ARTs," in *Cambridge Quarterly of Healthcare Ethics* 11, 4 (2002): 401–410.

HUMBER, James M. and ALMEDER, Robert F., *Reproduction, Technology, and Rights*, Humana Press, Totowa, NJ (1996).

HÜNERMANN, Peter (ed.), *Heinrich Denzinger, Compendium of Creeds, Definitions, and Declarations on Matters of Faith and Morals*: 3873a, 43rd Edition, Ignatius Press, San Francisco (2012).

JONSEN, Albert R., "Reproduction and Rationality," in *Cambridge Quarterly of Healthcare Ethics* 4, 3 (1995): 263–267.

KILNER, John F. (ed. et al.), *The Reproduction Revolution: A Christian Appraisal of Sexuality, Reproductive Technologies and the Family*, Eerdmans, Cambridge (2000).

LANGLOIS, Anne V., "Les nouvelles techniques de reproduction entre la loi et la morale," in Le *Supplement* 174 (1990): 29–34.

LYSAUGHT, Therese M., and KOTVA, Joseph Jr. (ed. et al.), *On Moral Medicine: Theological Perspectives in Medical Ethics*, 3rd edition, Grand Rapids, Cambridge (2012).

MACKLIN, Richard, "Artificial Means of Reproduction and Our Understanding of the Family," in *The Hastings Center Report* 21, 1 (1991): 5–11.

MAY, William E., *Marriage: The Rock on Which the Family Is Built*, Ignatius Press, San Francisco (1995).

———, *Catholic Bioethics and the Gift of Human Life*, 2nd edition, Our Sunday Visitor, Indiana (2008).

MAY, William E., LAWLER, Ronald and BOYLE, Joseph, Catholic Sexual Ethics: A Summary, Explanation, & Defense, 3rd edition, Our Sunday Visitor, Huntington (2011).

MCDONNEL, Orla, and ALLISON, Jill, "From Biopolitics to Bioethics: Church, State, Medicine and Assisted Reproductive Technology in Ireland," in *Sociology of Health and Illness* 28, 6 (2006): 817–837.

O'DONOVAN, Oliver, *Begotten or Made?* Reprint, Clarendon Press, Oxford (2002).

OVERALL, Christine, *Why Have Children? The Ethical Debate*, MIT Press, Massachusetts (2012).

PACE, Tyler N., *Bioethics: Issues and Dilemmas*. Hauppauge, Nova Science Publishers, New York (2010).

PAYNE, Franklin E., *Making Biblical Decisions*, Hosanna House, Escondido, CA (1989).

PUCA, Antonio, "Ten Years on From the Warnock Report: Is the Human Embryo a Person?" in *The Linacre Quarterly* 62, 2 (1995): 75–87.

RATZINGER, Joseph, "Uno sguardo teologico sulla procreazione umana," in *Medicina e Morale* 38 (1988): 507–521.

———, "Der Mensch Zwischen Reproduktion und Schöpfung: Theologische Fragen zum Ursprung des Menschlichen Lebens," in *Intern. Kath. Zeitschr. Communio*, t. 18 (1989): 61–71.

RHONHEIMER, Martin, *Etica della procreazione*, Pontificia Università Lateranense, Istituto Giovanni Paolo II, Roma (2000).

———, *Natural Law and Practical Reason: A Thomist View of Moral Autonomy*, English Translation, Gerald Malsbary, Fordham University Press, New York (2000).

RICHARD, Sparks C., "Helping Catholic Couples Conceive," April 1997, St. Anthony Messenger, www.americancatholic.org/apr1997/featurel.asp.

RODRÍQUEZ-LUÑO, Ángel, La dignità umana al centro della medicina: la vision cattolica, in *Medics* 13 (2005): 64–67.

———, *Scelti in Cristo per essere santi*, Vol. 3, EDUSC, Roma (2008).

RUSSO, Giovanni. *Dignitas personae: commenti all'Istruzione su alcune questioni di bioetica*, Coop. S. Tom, Messina (2009).

RYAN, Maura A., "Faith and Infertility," in M. Therese Lysaught and Joseph Kotva Jr. (ed. et al.), *On Moral Medicine: Theological Perspectives in Medical Ethics*, 3rd edition, Grand Rapids, Cambridge (2012): 865–869.

SAINT THOMAS AQUINAS, *Summa Theologiae: A Concise Translation*, edited by Timothy McDermott, Christian Classics, Westminster (1989).

SANDEL, Michael J., *The Case Against Perfection: Ethics in the Age of Genetic Engineering*, Harvard University Press, Massachusetts (2009).

SARMIENTO, Augusto, *La famiglia: futuro de la humanidad: documentos del magisterio de la iglesia*, Biblioteca de Autore Cristianos, Madrid (1995).

SCHLAG, Martin, *Das moralische Gesetz in Evangelium Vitae*, Peter Lang-Verlag, Frankfurt am Main (2000).

SCHUBERT, Von H., "Evangelische Ethik und Biotechnologie: Ein Bericht über die Deutschsprachige Diskussion," in *Zeitschr. Ev. Ethik* 35 (1991): 213–220.

SGRECCIA, Elio, *Manuale di bioetica: fondamenti ed Etica Biomedica*, 4th edition, V&P, Milano (2007).

———, *Personalist Bioethics*, English Trans. John A. Di Camillo and Michael J. Miller, The National Catholic Bioethics Center, Philadelphia (2012).

SHANNON, Thomas A., *The Nature and Dignity of the Human Person as the Foundation of the Right to Life: The Challenges of the Contemporary Cultural Context*, Libreria Editrice Vaticana, Vatican City 2002.

SHAPIRO, Donald E., *Birth, Law, Medicine and Morality*, Oxford Centre for Postgraduate Hebrew Studies, Oxford (1986).

———, "New Innovations in Conception and their Effects upon our Law and Morality," in *New York Law School law Review* 31, (1986): 37–59.

SINGER, Peter, and WELLS, Deane, *Making Babies: The New Science and Ethics of Conception*, C. Scribner's Sons, New York (1985).

SINGER, Peter, HELGE, Kuhse, BUCKLE, Stephen, DAWSON, Karen and KASIMBA, Pascal (eds.), *Embryo Experimentation*. Cambridge University Press, Cambridge (1990).

SMITH, George Patrick, *The Christian Religion and Biotechnology: A Search for Principled Decision-making*, Springer, Dordrecht, Norwell, MA (2005).

SMITH, Janet E., "The Vocation of Christian Marriage as an Approach to the Bioethics of Human Reproduction," in Marilyn Wallace and Thomas Hilgers (eds.), *The Gift of Life: The Proceedings of a National Conference on the Vatican Instruction on Reproductive Ethics and Technology*, Pope Paul VI Institute Press, Omaha, NE (1990): 49–60.

────── (ed.), *Why Humanae Vitae was Right: A Reader*, Ignatius Press, San Francisco (1993).

SMITH, Jennifer, "When Morality Gets in the Way: Public Policy Debates Around Reproductive Technologies," in *Just Policy: A Journal of Australian Social Policy* 38 (2005): 48–50.

SPAEMANN, Robert, *Die Unantastbarkeit Des Menschlichen Lebens: Zu Ethischen Fragen D. Biomedizin*, Herder, Freiburg (1987).

TAYLOR, Gordon, *The Biological Time Bomb*, New American Library, New York (1969).

TOLLESFSEN, Christopher, *John Paul II's Contribution to Catholic Bioethics*. Distributed in North, Central and South America by Springer, Dordrecht; Norwell, MA (2004).

VERHEY, Allen, "A.R.T, Ethics and the Bible," in M. Therese Lysaught and Joseph J. Kotva, Jr. (eds. et al.), *On Moral Medicine: Theological Perspectives in Medical Ethics*, 3rd edition, Grand Rapids, Cambridge (2012): 870–893.

VIAL CORREA, J. De D. and SGRECCIA, Elio (eds.), *Ethics of Biomedical Research: In a Christian Vision: Proceedings of the Ninth General Assembly of Pontifical Academy for Life*, Libreria Editrice Vaticana, Vatican City (2003).

WATT, Helen, "Parenthood and New Reproductive Technologies: Anthropological Considerations," in Juan De Dios Vial Correa and Elio Sgreccia (eds.), *The Dignity of Human Procreation and Reproductive Technologies: Anthropological and Ethical Aspects*, Libreria Vaticana, Vatican City (2005): 33–42.

WILDES, Kevin Wm (ed.), *Infertility: A Crossroad of Faith, Medicine, and Technology*, Kluwer Academic Publishers, Boston (1997).

WOJTYLA, Karol, *Amore e Responsabilità*, 3rd edition, Casa Editrice Marietti, Torino (1980).

www.ingramcontent.com/pod-product-compliance
Ingram Content Group UK Ltd.
Pitfield, Milton Keynes, MK11 3LW, UK
UKHW041438190426
11946UKWH00021B/12